WALKING NEW ORLEANS

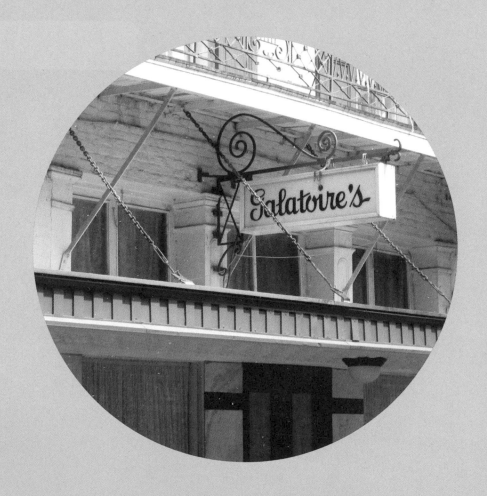

WALKING NEW ORLEANS

30 Tours Exploring Historic Neighborhoods, Waterfront Districts, Culinary and Music Corridors, and Recreational Wonderlands

Barri Bronston

 WILDERNESS PRESS . . . *on the trail since 1967*

Walking New Orleans: 30 Tours Exploring Historic Neighborhoods, Waterfront Districts, Culinary and Music Corridors, and Recreational Wonderlands

Copyright © 2015 by Barri Bronston

Project editor: Ritchey Halphen
Cover and interior photos: Copyright © by Barri Bronston, except where noted
Cartographer: Scott McGrew
Original cover and interior design: Larry B. Van Dyke and Lisa Pletka; typesetting and layout: Annie Long
Proofreader: Rebecca Benton Henderson
Indexer: Sylvia Coates

Cataloging-in-Publication Data is available from the Library of Congress.

ISBN: 978-0-89997-761-4; eISBN: 978-0-89997-762-1

Manufactured in the United States of America

Published by: **WILDERNESS PRESS**
An imprint of Keen Communications, LLC
PO Box 43673
Birmingham, AL 35243
800-443-7227; fax 205-326-1012

Visit **wildernesspress.com** for a complete listing of our books, and for ordering information. E-mail us at **info@wildernesspress.com** with questions or concerns.

Distributed by Publishers Group West

Cover photos: *Front, clockwise from bottom left:* Piety Street Arch, Crescent Park, Bywater; view of the Central Business District from the Algiers–Canal Street ferry landing, Algiers Point; Holocaust Memorial, Woldenberg Riverfront Park; Cresson House, Faubourg St. John; statues in Louis Armstrong Park, Treme. *Back, top to bottom:* Pat O'Brien's, French Quarter; Latter Memorial Library, St. Charles Avenue; Gumbel Memorial Fountain, Audubon Park.

Frontispiece: Galatoire's restaurant, Bourbon Street (see Walk 4, French Quarter)

SAFETY NOTICE Although Wilderness Press and the author have made every attempt to ensure that the information in this book is accurate at press time, they are not responsible for any loss, damage, injury, or inconvenience that may occur to anyone while using this book. You are responsible for your own safety and health while following the walking trips described here. Always check local conditions, know your own limitations, and consult a map.

acknowledgments

WRITING THIS BOOK WAS A CHALLENGING ENDEAVOR that I could not have fulfilled without the help of many individuals and organizations.

First of all, I would like to thank Wilderness Press for recognizing the importance of New Orleans as a walking city and former Acquisitions Editor Susan Haynes for giving me this amazing opportunity. I would also like to thank current Acquisitions Editor Tim Jackson for keeping me on track with deadlines and assisting with big-picture issues; Ritchey Halphen, a New Orleans native, for his amazing and meticulous editing; and the production team of cartographer Scott McGrew, typesetter Annie Long, proofreader Rebecca Henderson, and indexer Sylvia Coates for putting all the pieces together and adding the finishing touches.

In addition, I want to thank my sister Donna Goldenberg for her wonderful photography, along with her husband, Eric, and son, Trevor, who accompanied Donna and me on a walk through the breathtaking Jean Lafitte Barataria Preserve. And thanks to Janet Pesses for joining me on one of the longest walks in the book—that being the equally spectacular Lakefront area.

In addition, thanks go out to Kathryn Hobgood Ray for her help with the Algiers Point neighborhood, to Beth Donze for her expertise on Faubourg St. John, and to Lisanne Brown for steering me to Crescent Park and other funky spots in Bywater. A big thank-you to Eddie Bronston, my former husband but still good friend, for lending his musical expertise for the walk covering Faubourg Marigny and Frenchmen Street. I'd also like to acknowledge Mike Strecker, my boss at Tulane University, for reviewing the University section and making sure that I included some of Tulane's most important landmarks.

For two of the walks—the Lower Ninth Ward's Make It Right neighborhood and Jean Lafitte Barataria Preserve—I relied on their materials and maps, and for those I would like to thank both of them. I also want to thank the New Orleans Tourism Marketing Corporation and the St. Tammany Parish Tourist & Convention Commission for providing me with some terrific images.

Although she no longer lives in New Orleans—but knows it almost as well as I do—my daughter and best friend, Sally Bronston, served as a great sounding board as I pondered various aspects of the book, especially what bars and restaurants to include. Thanks, kid! You may live in New York City, but NOLA will always be home.   —*Barri Bronston*

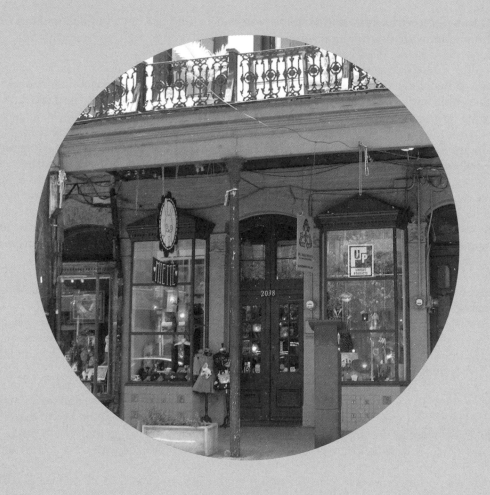

A stroll through the Lower Garden District (Walk 7) will take you past some of the funkiest shops on Magazine Street, including Miette, which sells locally made jewelry, clothing, and home accessories.

author's note

I WAS BORN IN NEW ORLEANS IN THE LATE 1950S, and except for four years attending college in Missouri and another year living in Arkansas, I've spent pretty much my entire life in what is often referred to as one of the world's most fascinating cities.

For most of that time, I was a journalist, an experience that gave me an up-close encounter with the people and places that have made New Orleans one of the coolest, craziest, and most captivating destinations on the map.

Still, as a native, I tended to take my city for granted. Not until I took on this book in the summer of 2013 did I really start to get it—that "it" being the heap of honors that have been bestowed on New Orleans in recent years, among them being named one of the world's top 10 cities by *Travel & Leisure,* a best American city for foodies by *Condé Nast Traveler,* and one of six trips that will change your life by *Coastal Living.* And in 2014, New Orleans came in seventh on the online magazine *Good*'s list of the 50 Most Inspiring Cities in the World—higher than any other city in the United States—based on its street vibrancy, green life, civic engagement, and entrepreneurship, among other factors.

The city has certainly overcome more than its fair share of challenges, but I'm more proud than ever to be a native and resident of New Orleans.

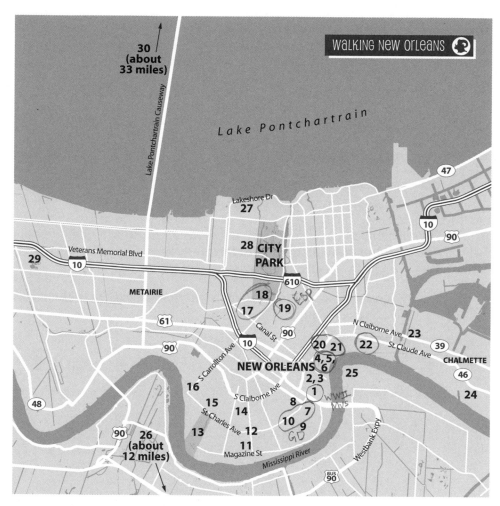

WALKING NEW ORLEANS

30
(about
33 miles)

Lake Pontchartrain Causeway

Lake Pontchartrain

47

Lakeshore Dr
27

28 CITY
PARK

610

29

Veterans Memorial Blvd

10

10

90

METAIRIE

18

17   19

ESP

61

90

Canal St

10

90

N Claiborne Ave   23

20 21   22   St Claude Ave   39

4, 5,

6   CHALMETTE

NEW ORLEANS   25   46

2, 3

16   S Claiborne Ave   1   WWII   24

48   15   S Charles Ave   8   MJs

14   7

13   12   10   9

26   11   GD

(about   Magazine St

12 miles)   Mississippi River   Westbank Expy

90   BUS
90

NUMBERS ON THIS LOCATOR MAP CORRESPOND TO WALK NUMBERS.

TABLE OF CONTENTS

INTRODUCTION

THE MANY RECENT ACCOLADES that New Orleans has received show just how far the city has come since August 29, 2005, when Hurricane Katrina became one of the most horrific disasters our country has ever known. That powerful, life-altering storm destroyed approximately 80 percent of New Orleans, killed more than 1,800 people, and forced hundreds of thousands to flee the city, some forever. Even worse, it had some politicians arguing against spending federal dollars to rebuild a city that lies 7 feet below sea level.

"It looks like a lot of that place could be bulldozed," then–Speaker of the House Dennis Hastert famously said just a few days after the storm.

There certainly was bulldozing to be done, but thankfully it was to make way for the rebuilding. That doesn't mean New Orleans has fully recovered—a decade later, some of the city's poorer neighborhoods continue to struggle—but overall, New Orleans is better than ever. Public education has improved, the movie business is booming, and in a city known for its dining scene, there are actually more restaurants today than there were before the storm.

There isn't a better way to see what all the fuss is about than by foot, be it through the historic Irish Channel, the funky Marigny, the colorful Bywater, or any of the other 27 walks in this book.

In big news for walkers, the Lafitte Greenway, a 2.6-mile multiuse trail and linear park, is scheduled to open in the spring of 2015. The greenway follows the route of the Lafitte Corridor, which was established as a shipping canal in the mid-1700s and later became a railway. A completed section of the greenway—which when finished will extend from Basin Street near the French Quarter to Canal Boulevard in the Lakeview neighborhood—is a point of interest in Walk 17, Mid-City (page 117).

New Orleans is far from utopic, and I struggled with whether or not to include some areas. I went back and forth with Treme, Oretha Castle Haley Boulevard, and even parts of the beloved French Quarter, but in the end I decided that there was too much historical significance and too many good things happening in these places to exclude them.　　*(continued)*

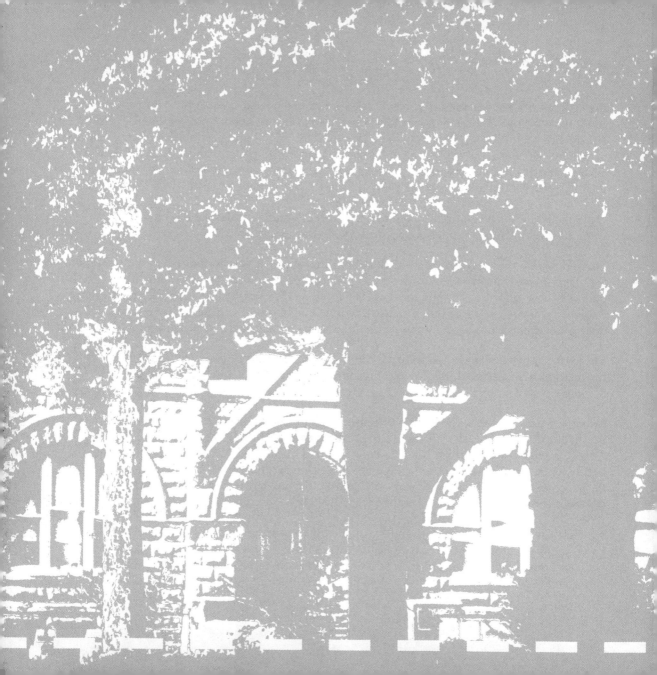

As you would on any walking tour, in any city, use common sense: Walk in groups, and avoid walking after dark. And as you're trekking away, be on the lookout for broken sidewalks and potholes, which sadly are common sights in many a New Orleans neighborhood.

Oh, and don't forget your water—especially if you plan to conquer one of these walks during the city's infamous sweltering summer.

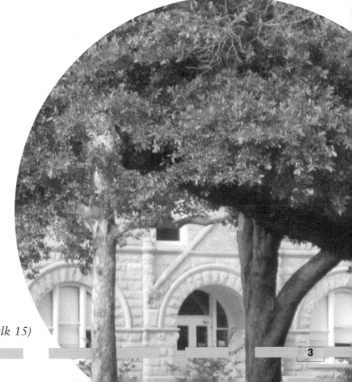

Gibson Hall, Tulane University (see Walk 15)

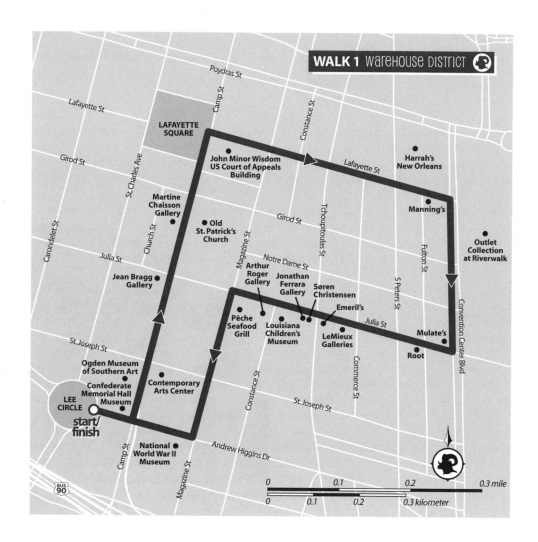

WALK 1 Warehouse District

Poydras St

Lafayette St

Girod St

Carondelet St

St. Charles Ave

Camp St

Church St

Magazine St

LAFAYETTE SQUARE

John Minor Wisdom US Court of Appeals Building

Lafayette St

Harrah's New Orleans

Constance St

Martine Chaisson Gallery

Manning's

Old St. Patrick's Church

Girod St

Tchoupitoulas St

Outlet Collection at Riverwalk

Fulton St

Julia St

Notre Dame St

Jean Bragg Gallery

Arthur Roger Gallery

Jonathan Ferrara Gallery

Søren Christensen

Emeril's

S Peters St

Convention Center Blvd

Pêche Seafood Grill

Louisiana Children's Museum

LeMieux Galleries

Julia St

Mulate's

St. Joseph St

Root

Ogden Museum of Southern Art

Confederate Memorial Hall Museum

Contemporary Arts Center

Commerce St

LEE CIRCLE

start/ finish

Constance St

St. Joseph St

Camp St

National World War II Museum

Andrew Higgins Dr

Magazine St

BUS 90

0   0.1   0.2   0.3 mile

0   0.1   0.2   0.3 kilometer

1 Warehouse District: an art Lover's paradise

BOUNDARIES: St. Charles Ave., Poydras St., Convention Center Blvd., Andrew Higgins Dr.
DISTANCE: 1.8 miles
PARKING: Lots, garages, metered parking
PUBLIC TRANSIT: St. Charles Ave. Streetcar

The Warehouse District, also called the Arts District, is by far one of the coolest neighborhoods in New Orleans, its establishment an answer to the urban blight that replaced a once-thriving industrial area. The Contemporary Arts Center pioneered the effort in 1976, converting a dilapidated building into a showcase for visual and performing artists.

Over the next quarter of a century, the area experienced a complete transformation, and today it is home to some of the city's preeminent museums, galleries, restaurants, and clubs. Countless buildings have been converted into luxury condo developments, making the Warehouse District one of the most desirable neighborhoods in town.

Museums include the National World War II Museum, the Ogden Museum of Southern Art, the Louisiana Children's Museum, and the Confederate Memorial Hall Museum. Julia Street boasts some of the city's top art galleries, among them the Arthur Roger Gallery, Jean Bragg Gallery, and Jonathan Ferrara Gallery.

The culinary scene is equally vibrant. Eateries range from upscale Emeril's and Tommy's to the trendy and hip Root and Pêche Seafood Grill. For drinks—and fun—gathering spots include Tommy's Wine Bar and Manning's, the sports bar and restaurant owned by Archie Manning, former New Orleans Saints quarterback and father of current NFL quarterbacks Eli and Peyton.

● Begin your walk at Lee Circle, where St. Charles Avenue intersects Andrew Higgins Drive. Lee Circle is known for its bronze statue of General Robert E. Lee, commander of the Confederate Army during the Civil War. The statue, which stands high atop a granite pedestal, was sculpted by Alexander Doyle in 1884.

● Walk a block down Andrew Higgins across Camp Street, and turn left. To the right is the Contemporary Arts Center, known for its bold, sometimes daring displays of

NATIONAL WORLD WAR II MUSEUM

When the National World War II Museum opened as the National D-Day Museum in 2000, there were just under 6 million surviving veterans of the so-called War That Changed the World. As of 2014, the number had dwindled to just over a million.

According to the Department of Veterans Affairs, veterans are dying at a rate of 550 a day, making the museum's mission—to ensure that all generations understand the price of freedom and be inspired by what they learn—that much more crucial.

Named by travel website TripAdvisor as a top-10 museum in the United States and the 14th best in the world, the National World War II Museum is fulfilling its mission through extraordinary exhibits that explain why the war was fought, how it was won, and what it means today.

The museum campus consists of three buildings, each dedicated to a central theme that gives visitors an opportunity to experience the war through the eyes of those who lived it. Exhibits include uniforms, weaponry, vehicles, medals, diaries, letters, artwork, photographs, and other mementos, along with oral histories and personal vignettes. The Solomon Victory Theater is home to the exclusive Tom Hanks production *Beyond All Boundaries,* a 4-D film that explains the war through dazzling special effects, archival footage, and first-person accounts. In December 2014, the museum opened its newest exhibit, "Road to Berlin: European Theater Galleries," a 32,000-square-foot multimedia experience that recounts the drama and personal sacrifices surrounding America's fight to defeat the Axis powers and preserve freedom.

Entertainment abounds as well, from Rat Pack tribute shows to performances by the Victory Belles, a 1940s-style singing group. And a program called White Glove Wednesdays invites visitors to try on original and reproduction helmets, uniforms, boots, packs, and other gear.

visual and performing arts. To the left is the Confederate Memorial Hall Museum, which houses artifacts from the Civil War, including the personal belongings of soldiers along with weapons, flags, and uniforms.

Adjacent to the Confederate Museum is the Ogden Museum of Southern Art, which showcases the visual arts of the American South, including the works of Clementine Hunter, George Dureau, and Ida Kohlmeyer. The museum, named after Southern art collector and philanthropist Roger Ogden, offers live music every Thursday night, film screenings related to Ogden's collections, and an impressive array of educational programming.

● Continue walking down Camp and cross St. Joseph Street. Halfway down the block to the left is Ozanam Inn, a nonprofit shelter and kitchen for the homeless. A program of the Society of St. Vincent de Paul, Ozanam works to help homeless individuals attain independence, offering medical treatment and legal counsel along with job and life-skills training.

At the corner of Camp and Julia Streets is one of the many art galleries that popu- late the Warehouse District, the Jean Bragg Gallery. Housed in an 1832 building listed on the National Register of Historic Places, the gallery showcases the works of Louisiana artists, both new and established. Among its specialties are Newcomb and Gulf Coast pottery.

● Cross Julia and continue walking down Camp. On the left is the Martine Chaisson Gallery, which, like so many of the galleries in the Warehouse District, represents both emerging and established contemporary artists. Toward the end of the block, to the right, is the Old St. Patrick's Church, which is also on the National Register of Historic Places. The church celebrated its first Mass in 1840. At the time, services took place in a small wooden structure. Longing to worship in the same splendor that the French citizenry did at nearby St. Louis Cathedral, the Irish community rallied support for its own house of worship, and the Gothic-style Old St. Patrick's was born.

Two blocks past St. Patrick's is the John Minor Wisdom US Court of Appeals Building, headquarters of the Fifth Circuit Court of Appeals, which hears cases from Louisiana, Texas, and Mississippi. Built in 1915 in the Italian Renaissance Revival style, the three-story marble-and-granite building features a cornice inscribed with the names of former chief justices of the US Supreme Court. The building is named for John Minor Wisdom, who served on the appellate court from 1957 until his death in 1999.

Wisdom was a highly respected judge who promoted civil rights through landmark decisions involving school desegregation and voter rights.

Directly across from the courthouse is Lafayette Square, the second oldest park in New Orleans. The park features several statues, including one of John McDonogh, the founder of the city's school system. From March to June, the park is home to the weekly "Wednesdays in the Square," a concert series sponsored by the Young Leadership Council.

Look across the square and you'll see Gallier Hall, one of New Orleans's most iconic landmarks. Dedicated in 1853, the Greek Revival structure served as City Hall for a century and continues today as a special-events venue and occasional set location for movies and TV shows, including *NCIS: New Orleans.* On Mardi Gras Day, the mayor of New Orleans toasts the kings of the Zulu and Rex parades here.

● Turn right on Lafayette Street and walk seven blocks to Convention Center Boulevard. This stretch will take you behind the Hale Boggs Federal Building and Courthouse to Fulton Street, a block-long entertainment mall featuring an array of restaurants and bars. Every winter, Harrah's New Orleans presents "Miracle on Fulton Street," converting the walkway into a wonderland of lights, decorations, and snowfall. Among the restaurants on Fulton is Manning's, an upscale sports bar owned by former New Orleans Saints quarterback Archie Manning in partnership with Harrah's. The restaurant features 30 flat-screen TVs, a sports-anchor desk, and memorabilia from Louisiana's first family of football—Archie and sons Peyton and Eli—and various Louisiana teams. A row of comfy recliners faces the bar's mega-screen.

● At Convention Center Boulevard, turn right and walk three blocks to Julia Street. Across the boulevard is the Outlet Collection at Riverwalk, a high-end outlet mall, and the Ernest N. Morial Convention Center, named after the first black mayor of New Orleans. At 1.1 million square feet, the center is the sixth largest in the United States.

● Turn right on Julia at Mulate's, a popular Cajun restaurant where you can try such Louisiana fare as fried alligator and stuffed catfish, as well as test your Cajun two-step skills on the dance floor.

- From Mulate's, walk six blocks down Julia to Magazine Street. This stretch features some of the city's most respected art galleries, among them LeMieux Galleries, Søren Christensen, Jonathan Ferrara Gallery, and Arthur Roger Gallery. All invite visitors to stop in and browse. Julia Street is the center of two of the most popular arts events in town—White Linen Night and Art for Arts' Sake. The galleries also present Art Walks on the first Saturday night of every month.

  Restaurants also abound on Julia, including Emeril's New Orleans, the flagship restaurant of celebrity chef Emeril Lagasse, at the corner of Tchoupitoulas Street. Other restaurants along Julia or in the general vicinity are Root, Tomas Bistro, Tommy's Cuisine, and Tommy's Wine Bar.

  At the corner of Julia and Constance Streets is the Louisiana Children's Museum, which promotes learning through such exhibits as the Little Port of New Orleans, Art Trek, and the Little Winn-Dixie Grocery Store. At the Louisiana Hospitality Foundation Kids' Café, children learn about the city's restaurant industry by playing the roles of server, cook, and maître d'. Long-term plans call for the museum to move to City Park, providing it with an outdoor learning space.

- Turn left on Magazine Street. To the left is Pêche Seafood Grill, which, since opening to rave reviews in 2013, has become one of the city's most talked-about dining spots. In May 2014, it won the James Beard Award for the Best New Restaurant in America, beating out three restaurants in New York and one in San Francisco.

- Walk two blocks to Andrew Higgins Drive, home of the National World War II Museum (see sidebar). Through interactive exhibits, oral histories, and vignettes, the museum tells the story of the so-called War That Changed the World. The museum's Stage Door Canteen presents war-era entertainment from big-band favorites to the Victory Belles singing group (think the Andrews Sisters).

- Turn right at Andrew Higgins and head two blocks back to Lee Circle.

POINTS OF INTEREST

Robert E. Lee Monument St. Charles Avenue at Lee Circle

Confederate Memorial Hall Museum confederatemuseum.com, 922 Camp St., 504-523-4522

Contemporary Arts Center cacno.org, 900 Camp St., 504-528-3805

Ogden Museum of Southern Art ogdenmuseum.org, 925 Camp St., 504-539-9650

Jean Bragg Gallery jeanbragg.com 600 Julia St., 504-895-7375

Old St. Patrick's Church oldstpatricks.org, 724 Camp St., 504-525-4413

Martine Chaisson Gallery martinechaissongallery.com, 727 Camp St., 504-302-7942

Old St. Patrick's Church oldstpatricks.org, 724 Camp St., 504-525-4413

John Minor Wisdom US Court of Appeals Building tinyurl.com/jmwbuilding, 600 Camp St., 504-310-7700

Lafayette Square nola.gov/parks-and-parkways/parks-squares/lafayette-square, bounded by St. Charles Ave., Camp St., N. Maestri St., and S. Maestri St.; 504-658-3200

Manning's harrahsneworleans.com/restaurants.html, 519 Fulton St., 504-593-8118

Outlet Collection at Riverwalk riverwalkneworleans.com, 500 Port of New Orleans, 504-522-1555

Mulate's mulates.com, 201 Julia St., 504-522-1492

Root rootnola.com, 200 Julia St., 504-252-9480

Emeril's emerilsrestaurants.com, 800 Tchoupitoulas St., 504-528-9393

LeMieux Galleries lemieuxgalleries.com, 332 Julia St., 504-522-5988

Søren Christensen sorengallery.com, 400 Julia St., 504-569-9501

Jonathan Ferrara Gallery jonathanferraragallery.com, 400-A Julia St., 504-522-5471

Louisiana Children's Museum lcm.org, 420 Julia St., 504-523-1357

Arthur Roger Gallery arthurrogergallery.com, 432 Julia St., 504-522-1999

Pêche Seafood Grill pecherestaurant.com, 800 Magazine St., 504-522-1744

National World War II Museum nationalww2museum.org, 945 Magazine St., 504-527-6012

route summary

1. Begin at Lee Circle and Andrew Higgins Drive.
2. Walk one block to Camp Street; cross Camp and turn left.
3. Walk five blocks to Lafayette Street and turn right.
4. Walk seven blocks to Convention Center Boulevard and turn right.
5. Walk three blocks to Julia Street and turn right.
6. Walk six blocks to Magazine Street and turn left.
7. Walk two blocks to Andrew Higgins and turn right.
8. Walk two blocks to Lee Circle.

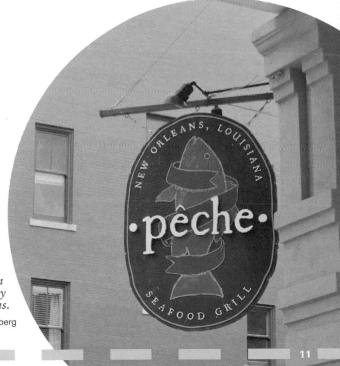

Pêche Seafood Grill, known for its vast selection of coastal seafood, is an essential stop for any foodie traveling to New Orleans.

Photo: Donna Goldenberg

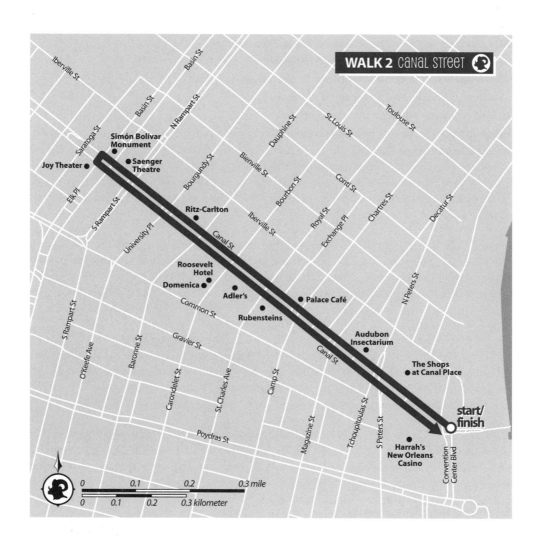

Iberville St

Basin St

Basin St

N Rampart St

Saratoga St

Simón Bolívar
Monument

Dauphine St

St. Louis St

Toulouse St

Joy Theater

Saenger
Theatre

Bourgundy St

Bienville St

Bourbon St

Conti St

Chartres St

Decatur St

Elk Pl

S Rampart St

Ritz-Carlton

Iberville St

Royal St

Exchange Pl

University Pl

Canal St

Roosevelt
Hotel

Domenica

Adler's

Palace Café

N Peters St

Common St

Rubensteins

Audubon
Insectarium

S Rampart St

Gravier St

Canal St

The Shops
at Canal Place

O'Keefe Ave

Barone St

Carondelet St

St. Charles Ave

Camp St

Magazine St

Tchoupitoulas St

S Peters St

start/
finish

Poydras St

Harrah's
New Orleans
Casino

Convention Center Blvd

0   0.1   0.2   0.3 mile

0   0.1   0.2   0.3 kilometer

2 Canal Street: revival in progress

BOUNDARIES: Canal St., Basin St., Convention Center Blvd.
DISTANCE: 1.93 miles
PARKING: Lots, garages, metered parking
PUBLIC TRANSIT: St. Charles Ave. Streetcar

Ask older natives of New Orleans about their memories of Canal Street, and you'll likely see their eyes light up as they recall dressing up in their finest attire and heading downtown to what was once the city's equivalent of Fifth Avenue. Back in the day, Canal Street—named for a canal that was never built—was the city's primary shopping destination, home to such classic department stores as Gus Mayer, Godchaux's, Kreeger's, Holmes, Krauss, and Maison Blanche.

As enclosed shopping malls began sprouting up in the suburbs and many of these stores began opening multiple locations, Canal—which separates the French Quarter from the Central Business District—took a major hit. Crowds began to thin, opting for the convenience of the malls, near which New Orleanians were moving in droves. By the late 1990s, only a couple of specialty stores, Adler's and Rubenstein Bros., remained.

To be sure, Canal Street was not the same—not that it had turned into a ghost town, but the quality of the shopping had been reduced to fast-food restaurants and discount stores peddling electronics, souvenirs, and T-shirts. Today, many of those outlets still exist, but a major revitalization effort has made Canal Street a destination once again, with upscale stores, luxury hotels and apartments, theaters, and restaurants now in the mix.

- **Begin at 333 Canal Street, home of The Shops at Canal Place and the Westin Hotel New Orleans. Stores at Canal Place include Saks Fifth Avenue, Brooks Brothers, and Tiffany and Co. The complex also features a luxury nine-screen movie theater, where you can dine on gourmet goodies from chef Adolfo Garcia's Gusto in the comfort of plush stadium-style seating.**

- **Walk one block. Between North Peters and Decatur Streets is the Audubon Butterfly Garden and Insectarium, one of the many museums of the Audubon Institute.**

Located in the historic US Custom House, it is the largest free-standing museum dedicated to insects in North America. Highlights include a butterfly exhibit in an Asian-inspired garden, a hilarious animated-bug movie featuring the voices of Joan Rivers and Brad Garrett, and up-close encounters with cockroaches, ants, and other creatures you love to hate. At the Bug Appetite Buffet, you can sample bug-inspired treats such as six-legged salsa and chocolate chirp cookies. Yes, the ingredients include edible insects.

● Continue down Canal Street just past Chartres Street, where you'll see the Palace Café, a Brennan family restaurant known for such contemporary Creole dishes as crabmeat cheesecake, duck-and-roasted-garlic gumbo, and white-chocolate bread pudding. The restaurant is housed in another historic structure: the old Werlein's Building, which until 1990 was one of *the* places in New Orleans to buy sheet music, pianos, and other musical instruments.

● As you continue walking down Canal Street, you'll pass several luxury hotels, including the Ritz-Carlton, where jazz favorite Jeremy Davenport performs regularly in the Davenport Lounge. The Ritz opened in 2000 in what was once the headquarters of Maison Blanche, one of the city's most popular department stores. Similarly, the Hyatt French Quarter is housed in the old D. H. Holmes building. Holmes, another of New Orleans's legendary department stores, was known as much for its exterior clock as it was for its merchandise. If you were meeting friends downtown, you likely were meeting them "under the clock at D. H. Holmes"—a location immortalized in *A Confederacy of Dunces,* the beloved comic novel by John Kennedy Toole.

● Walk two blocks and cross North Rampart Street. To the right is the venerable Saenger Theatre, home to the Broadway in New Orleans series. Listed on the National Register of Historic Places, the Saenger opened in 1927 as a venue for silent movies and stage shows. The theater's trademark feature was its European-style interior, designed by architect Emile Weil to resemble an Italian Baroque courtyard. As part of the design, Weil installed dozens of tiny lights in the ceiling, arranging them as constellations of the night sky. The design made the Saenger the South's grandest theater and the city's preeminent place to experience "moving pictures." In 2005, the Saenger was destroyed by Hurricane Katrina, the storm's floodwaters and winds causing millions of dollars in damage. The Broadway series moved to the nearby

Mahalia Jackson Theatre for the Performing Arts, where it remained until September 2013 when the Saenger unveiled its magnificent renovated digs. Costing an estimated $53 million, the restoration combines the grandness of the past with state-of-the-art performance features such as an updated orchestra pit, a deeper stage, and first-class sound and lighting systems. The rebirth of the Saenger is considered a major step in the revitalization of Canal Street.

● One block past the Saenger, on your right as you approach the intersection of Canal and Basin Streets, note the statue of Venezuelan military and political giant Simón Bolívar, who led the fight for Latin American independence from Spain in the 1800s. The 12-foot-high cast-granite statue is one of three monuments to Central and South American heroes that make up the Garden of the Americas, which honors the ties between New Orleans and Latin America. The other statues are of Mexican statesman Benito Juárez (Basin and Conti), who lived in Faubourg Marigny (see Walk 21) during the 1840s, and Francisco Morazán (Basin and St. Louis), who served as president of the Federal Republic of Central America—which comprised present-day Costa Rica, El Salvador, Guatemala, Honduras, and Nicaragua—from 1830 to 1839.

● Just past the monument, at 1201 Canal, is yet another former retail outlet: the site of Krauss Company, once the largest department store in the South. Now a luxury condominium development, Krauss closed in 1997, leaving behind a legacy of faithful shoppers who relished the store's old-fashioned ways of doing business. In addition to being the first store in the city to install air-conditioning and escalators (known as mechanical stairways), Krauss boasted such departments as notions, fabrics, and foundations, along with a lunch counter that served New Orleans cuisine.

● Cross Canal at Basin Street. The center of Canal—which like all medians in New Orleans is called the neutral ground—is where streetcars pass, so be extra-cautious as you walk to the other side of the street. At Canal and Basin is the Joy Theater, another of the city's longtime entertainment venues. Opened in 1947 as a movie house, it was one of four movie theaters (along with the Orpheum, State Palace, and Saenger) that populated downtown. Faced with growing competition from multi-theater complexes with stadium seating, the Joy shut down in 2003. It remained closed until 2011, when it reopened as a state-of-the-art venue for live music, theatrical performances, and other special events.

- From the Joy, continue walking down Canal Street toward the river. Walk three blocks to University Place. The 121-year-old Roosevelt Hotel, just off Canal Street, is well worth a side visit, especially during December, when its grand block-long lobby is converted to a winter wonderland complete with thousands of twinkling lights, a New Orleans–themed gingerbread village, and a white-birch canopy. In addition, the hotel is home to the famed Sazerac Bar and the wildly popular Domenica, a contemporary Italian restaurant that *Travel & Leisure* magazine in 2012 named one of the best Italian eateries in the country. Like so many of the city's historic buildings, the luxury hotel sustained extensive damage from Hurricane Katrina, and restoring it cost nearly $150 million. When it reopened in 2009 as part of the Waldorf Astoria hotel group, it won rave reviews from critics and guests alike.

- As you continue down Canal, you'll notice numerous chain stores, many of which occupy the spaces that once housed some of the city's premiere department stores. Sports Plus, at 828 Canal, is housed in the old Godchaux's building. CVS, at 800 Canal, was once Gus Mayer. In the middle of the block, at 824 Canal, is the home of the Boston Club, probably the city's most exclusive men's social club. Many of its members belong to blue-blood Carnival groups such as Rex and Comus. Until 1992, Rex, King of Carnival, toasted the Queen of Carnival at reviewing stands erected outside the Boston Club on Mardi Gras Day. That royal tradition now takes place outside the nearby Hotel InterContinental.

  At 772 Canal Street is Adler's, the city's oldest jewelry store. Adler's opened in 1898 in the French Quarter but outgrew that location and eventually moved to Canal. Even when their retail neighbors were closing up shop, Adler's never gave up on Canal. Neither did nearby Rubenstein Bros., an upscale men's clothing store that opened at the corner of Canal and St. Charles in 1924 and continues to thrive today as Rubensteins.

- Continue walking down Canal Street past Rubensteins and various other shops and hotels. The walk ends at Harrah's New Orleans Casino, at the corner of Canal and Convention Center Boulevard.

POINTS OF INTEREST

The Shops at Canal Place theshopsatcanalplace.com, 333 Canal St., 504-522-9200

Audubon Insectarium auduboninstitute.org/visit/insectarium, 423 Canal St., 504-524-2847

Palace Café palacecafe.com, 605 Canal St., 504-523-1661

Saenger Theatre saengernola.com, 1111 Canal St., 504-525-1052

Joy Theater thejoytheater.com, 1200 Canal St., 504-528-9569

Roosevelt Hotel therooseveltneworleans, 130 Roosevelt Way, 504-648-1200

Domenica domenicarestaurant.com, 123 Baronne St., 504-648-6020

Adler's adlersjewelry.com, 722 Canal St., 504-523-5292

Rubensteins rubensteinsneworleans.com, 102 St. Charles Ave., 504-581-6666

Harrah's New Orleans harrahsneworleans.com, 228 Poydras St.,
    800-427-7247

ROUTE SUMMARY

1. Begin walk at The Shops at Canal Place.
2. Walk 11 blocks to Basin Street.
3. Cross Canal at Basin and turn left.
4. Walk 11 blocks on the opposite side of Canal to Harrah's New Orleans Casino.

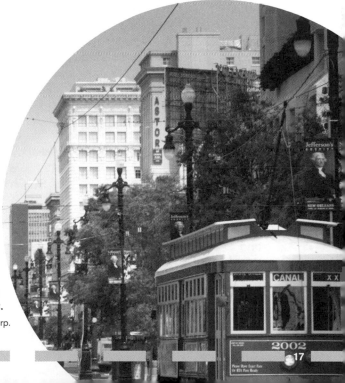

Canal Street, once the city's premiere shopping destination, is making a steady comeback, thanks to the efforts of the nonprofit Canal Street Redevelopment Corporation.

Photo courtesy of New Orleans Tourism Marketing Corp.

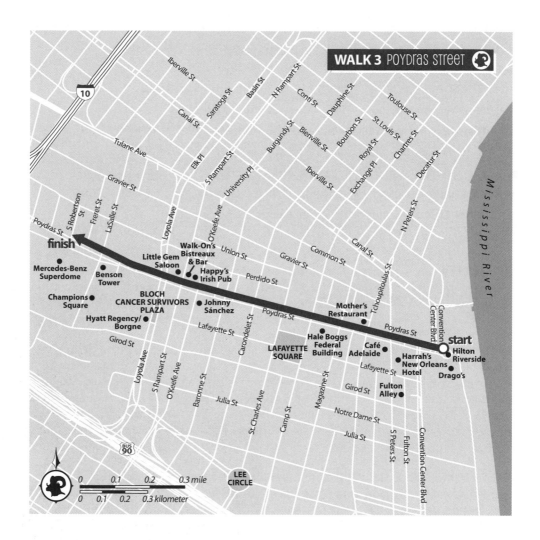

Iberville St

Saratoga St

Basin St

N Rampart St

Conti St

Dauphine St

Toulouse St

10

Canal St

Tulane Ave

Burgundy St

Bienville St

Bourbon St

St. Louis St

Chartres St

Gravier St

Elk Pl

S Rampart St

University Pl

Iberville St

Royal St

Exchange Pl

Decatur St

S Robertson St

Freret St

LaSalle St

Loyola Ave

O'Keefe Ave

N Peters St

Poydras St

finish

Walk-On's
Bistreaux
& Bar

Union St

Gravier St

Common St

Canal St

Mississippi River

Little Gem
Saloon

Happy's
Irish Pub

Mercedes-Benz
Superdome

Benson
Tower

Perdido St

Champions
Square

BLOCH
CANCER SURVIVORS
PLAZA

Johnny
Sánchez

Poydras St

Mother's
Restaurant

Tchoupitoulas St

Poydras St

Convention Center Blvd

start

Hyatt Regency/
Borgne

Lafayette St

Hilton
Riverside

Girod St

LAFAYETTE
SQUARE

Hale Boggs
Federal
Building

Café
Adelaide

Harrah's
New Orleans
Hotel

Drago's

Loyola Ave

S Rampart St

O'Keefe Ave

Baronne St

Carondelet St

Lafayette St

Magazine St

Girod St

Fulton
Alley

Julia St

St. Charles Ave

Camp St

Notre Dame St

Julia St

S Peters St

Fulton St

Convention Center Blvd

BUS
90

LEE
CIRCLE

0   0.1   0.2   0.3 mile

0   0.1   0.2   0.3 kilometer

3 POYDRAS STREET: SKYSCRAPER CENTRAL

BOUNDARIES: **Mississippi River, Poydras St., S. Robertson St.**
DISTANCE: **2.04 miles**
PARKING: **Lots, garages, metered parking**
PUBLIC TRANSIT: **Riverfront Streetcar, St. Charles Ave. Streetcar**

Poydras Street, the main thoroughfare of the Central Business District, extends from the Mississippi River to well beyond downtown. But it's the stretch between the river and South Claiborne Avenue that serves as the heartbeat of the city's economy, with the Mercedes-Benz Superdome anchoring one side and the busy riverfront and the nearby Ernest N. Morial Convention Center the other.

Poydras Street is named after Julien Poydras, a French-American politician who represented Louisiana in the US House of Representatives from 1809 to 1811. Until the oil boom of the 1980s, Poydras was just another downtown street, consisting mostly of low- to mid-rise buildings. But with the construction of the Superdome in 1975, along with such buildings as One Shell Square—the city's tallest—and 1250 Poydras Plaza, the city's skyline began taking shape. Although Poydras lost many tenants to the oil bust in the late '80s, many buildings were converted into luxury hotels to accommodate the city's ever-growing tourist industry.

Other high-rises on Poydras include the Pan American Life Center, Benson Tower, and First Bank and Trust Tower. Several hotels, restaurants, and bars can also be found on Poydras and in the surrounding business district, making New Orleans an ideal choice for conventions and big-time events such as the Super Bowl and the NCAA's Final Four. A relatively recent addition to the street is the Poydras Corridor Sculpture Exhibition, featuring more than a dozen sculptures by Southern artists, on the neutral ground between the Superdome and Convention Center Boulevard.

● **Begin at the Hilton New Orleans Riverside and cross Poydras Street. The vacant high-rise in front of you was once home to the World Trade Center of New Orleans and headquarters of the Port of New Orleans. Built in 1968, the 33-story structure housed foreign consulates and featured a popular revolving bar that overlooked the**

Mississippi River. The Port has since moved its offices to the riverfront, and the city is looking to repurpose the building as mixed commercial and residential space.

- Turn left and continue down Poydras in front of Harrah's, the city's only land-based casino. At 115,000 square feet, it has more than 1,800 slot machines, over 90 table games, and a concert venue. It's also the home of Besh Steak, one of eight eateries in celebrity chef John Besh's restaurant empire.

- A block from Harrah's, at Poydras and Tchoupitoulas Streets, is Mother's Restaurant, a po'boy joint that attracts huge lunch crowds. For the uninitiated, po'boys are similar to submarine sandwiches but are made on Louisiana's famous crisp French bread. At one time, Mother's was *the* quintessential spot to grab a sloppy roast beef or fried shrimp, and while it's still worth the stop, po'boys of all sizes, fillings, and prices abound across the metro area.

- Along Poydras Street, you'll pass numerous hotels and skyscrapers, including One Shell Square, between St. Charles Avenue and Carondelet Street. At 51 stories, One Shell Square is the tallest building in New Orleans and Louisiana. When it was built in 1972, it was also the tallest building in the Southeast, and the first Southern skyscraper to exceed 600 feet.

  Between South Rampart Street and O'Keefe Avenue sits a mini–entertainment area featuring Walk-On's Bistreaux & Bar, Happy's Irish Pub, and Little Gem Saloon, one of the city's newest music venues. Little Gem has an especially fascinating history: The club actually dates back to 1904, when it served as a popular hangout for such jazz legends as Jelly Roll Morton and Buddy Bolden. It closed in 1909, and though several other businesses occupied the space over the years, the building sat dormant for nearly 40 years until a group of developers and jazz aficionados brought it back to life as Little Gem in 2012. Regular performers include Dr. Michael White's Quartet, Kermit Ruffins and the Barbecue Swingers, Trombone Shorty, and the Viper Mad Trio.

- Cross Loyola Avenue and continue walking along Poydras, past the back of New Orleans City Hall and several other buildings, including 1555 Poydras, one of many buildings that make up Tulane University's downtown Health Sciences Campus.

- Make a left across Poydras at South Robertson Street, and take in the wonder that is the Mercedes-Benz Superdome, among the most recognizable structures in

New Orleans. Home of the New Orleans Saints since 1975, the Superdome is also home to the annual Allstate Sugar Bowl; the R&L Carriers New Orleans Bowl; the Bayou Classic; and the Essence Festival, the world's largest African American music festival. Over the years, it has undergone numerous facelifts, but none as sizable as the one following Hurricane Katrina in August 2005, when the Superdome served as a last-resort shelter for thousands of evacuees. The powerful storm peeled off part of the roof, and the damage from flooding was so extensive that the building had to be shut down for more than a year for repairs. That year, the Saints played their home games at Tiger Stadium in Baton Rouge, about 90 miles upriver from New Orleans. The Superdome reopened to much fanfare in September 2006, when the Saints beat the Atlanta Falcons in a nationally televised prime-time game.

● Continue walking down Poydras to LaSalle Street. To the right, down LaSalle, is Champions Square, a festival and concert venue built after the Saints won the Super Bowl in 2010. Saints fans, donning their black and gold, enjoy partying at the Square before each home game.

● Across from the Superdome is the 26-story Benson Tower, an office building owned by Saints and New Orleans Pelicans owner Tom Benson. The Hyatt Regency New Orleans, which was shuttered for six years after Katrina, is on that same block. The Hyatt is home to Borgne, another of John Besh's popular restaurants. As of this writing, plans were under way to convert a parking lot at the corner of Poydras and Loyola Avenue into an entertainment complex anchored by a 40,000-square-foot Dave & Buster's restaurant and arcade.

● Cross Loyola. To the right, on the median, is the Richard and Annette Bloch Cancer Survivors Plaza, one of two dozen parks around the country established by Richard Bloch, cofounder of H&R Block and a cancer survivor himself until his death from heart failure in 2004. The building at Loyola and Poydras is the Energy Centre, which at 39 stories is the city's fourth-tallest structure.

Between O'Keefe Avenue and Baronne Street, you'll pass a strip that includes several restaurants, among them Horinoya, serving Japanese cuisine; Reginelli's Pizzeria; and a Jimmy John's sandwich shop that's part of a franchise owned by Saints quarterback Drew Brees. The newcomer to the block is Johnny Sánchez, a taqueria co-owned by John Besh and Mexican American chef Aarón Sánchez, a regular judge on *Chopped* on the Food Network. The restaurant opened in the fall of 2014.

It's not included in this tour because of ongoing construction, but the South Market District, a redevelopment project two blocks off Poydras between Baronne Street and Loyola Avenue, promises to transform a barren part of the Central Business District into a spectacular complex of luxury apartments, entertainment venues, restaurants, and shops.

● Walk six blocks to Camp Street. The Hale Boggs Federal Building and Courthouse takes up the block between Camp and Magazine. New Orleans has long been known as a hotbed of political corruption, and this is where many elected officials, including former Louisiana governor Edwin Edwards, met their fates.

Three blocks from the Courthouse, between Tchoupitoulas and St. Peter Streets, is the Piazza d'Italia, built in the late 1970s as a monument to the city's Italian American community. At the Loews New Orleans Hotel, in the same block, is one of the Brennan family's top-rated restaurants, Café Adelaide. The eatery is named for the late Adelaide Brennan, a hat-loving, larger-than-life Auntie Mame type. On Saturdays and Sundays, "Brunch with Hat-itude" includes three free martinis (or "hat"-tinis) for those who don hats. (Baseball caps don't count.)

● Walk another block to Fulton Street. Closed to traffic, Fulton is an entertainment mall featuring such restaurants as Grand Isle and Ruth's Chris Steak House, along with the upscale bowling alley—yes, upscale—Fulton Alley. Every winter, Harrah's New Orleans Casino presents "Miracle on Fulton Street," converting the walkway into a wonderland of lights, decorations, and snowfall.

● Walk another block to Convention Center Boulevard and back to the Hilton. If you're hungry, grab a bite at Drago's Seafood, an iconic restaurant famous for its succulent chargrilled oysters.

POINTS OF INTEREST

Harrah's New Orleans harrahsneworleans.com, 228 Poydras St., 800-427-7247

Mother's Restaurant mothersrestaurant.net, 401 Poydras St., 504-523-9656

Happy's Irish Pub happysirishpub.com, 1009 Poydras St., 504-304-9236

Walk-On's Bistreaux & Bar walk-ons.com, 1009 Poydras St., 504-309-6530

Little Gem Saloon littlegemsaloon.com, 445 S. Rampart St., 504-267-4863

Mercedes-Benz Superdome superdome.com, 1500 Sugar Bowl Drive, 504-587-3663

Borgne borgnerestaurant.com, 601 Loyola Ave., 504-613-3860

Johnny Sánchez New Orleans johnnysanchezrestaurant.com, 930 Poydras St., 504-304-6615

Café Adelaide cafeadelaide.com, 300 Poydras St., 504-595-3305

Grand Isle Restaurant grandislerestaurant.com, 575 Convention Center Blvd., 504-520-8540

Ruth's Chris Steak House ruthschris.com, 525 Fulton St., 504-587-7099

Fulton Alley fultonalley.com, 600 Fulton St., 504-208-5569

Drago's Seafood Restaurant dragosrestau rant.com, 2 Poydras St., 504-584-3911

ROUTE SUMMARY

1. Begin walk at the Hilton Riverside hotel.
2. Cross Poydras Street and turn left.
3. Walk 16 blocks down Poydras to South Robertson Street.
4. Turn left to cross Poydras.
5. Walk 16 blocks back down Poydras to the Hilton Riverside.

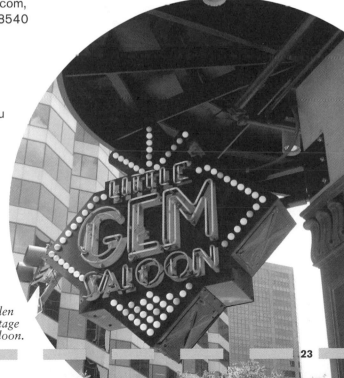

Jazz musicians Kermit Ruffins and Shamarr Allen are among the regular performers gracing the stage at the Little Gem Saloon.

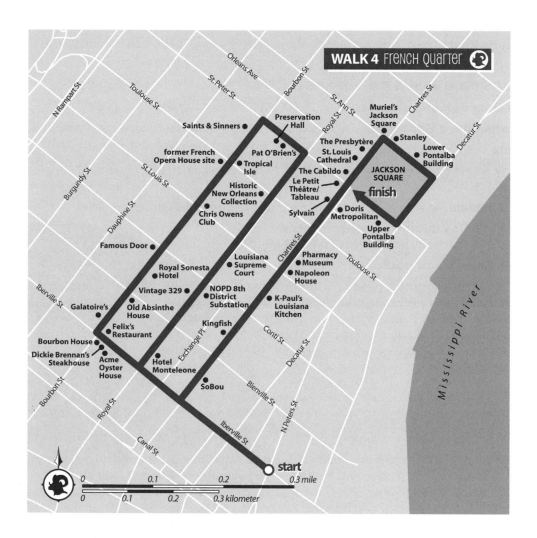

Orleans Ave

St. Peter St

Toulouse St

N Rampart St

Bourbon St

St. Ann St

Chartres St

Royal St

Decatur St

St. Louis St

Burgundy St

Dauphine St

Saints & Sinners

Preservation Hall

Muriel's Jackson Square

Stanley

former French Opera House site

Pat O'Brien's

The Presbytère

Lower Pontalba Building

Tropical Isle

St. Louis Cathedral

Historic New Orleans Collection

The Cabildo

JACKSON SQUARE

Le Petit Théâtre/ Tableau

finish

Chris Owens Club

Sylvain

Doris Metropolitan

Upper Pontalba Building

Famous Door

Louisiana Supreme Court

Pharmacy Museum

Toulouse St

Royal Sonesta Hotel

Napoleon House

Mississippi River

Vintage 329

NOPD 8th District Substation

K-Paul's Louisiana Kitchen

Iberville St

Galatoire's

Old Absinthe House

Kingfish

Chartres St

Conti St

Decatur St

Felix's Restaurant

Bourbon House

Dickie Brennan's Steakhouse

Acme Oyster House

Hotel Monteleone

SoBou

Bienville St

N Peters St

Exchange Pl

Bourbon St

Royal St

Iberville St

Canal St

start

0   0.1   0.2   0.3 mile

0   0.1   0.2   0.3 kilometer

4 French Quarter: Where History Meets Fun

BOUNDARIES: **Iberville St., Bourbon St., St. Ann St., Decatur St.**
DISTANCE: **1.66 miles**
PARKING: **Several garages and lots along N. Peters St.**
PUBLIC TRANSIT: **Riverfront Streetcar, St. Charles Ave. Streetcar**

To much of the outside world, the French Quarter is synonymous with Bourbon Street, that often sleazy yet strangely magical playground where you can let loose with a Hurricane or a Hand Grenade, go crazy for a pair of beads, or party so hard that when you wake up the next day, you just might wonder who you are and where you've been.

But the French Quarter, or the Vieux Carré, as it's known in French, is a hotbed of fascinating history, culinary artistry, and mesmerizing music. It's the antiques shops of Royal Street, the artists of Jackson Square, and the jazz musicians of Preservation Hall. It's Friday lunch at Galatoire's or late-night drinks at the Napoleon House.

The French Quarter is the oldest neighborhood in New Orleans, developed after the city's founding in 1718 by Jean-Baptiste Le Moyne de Bienville. Most of the historic buildings in the Quarter were built in the late 18th century, after two devastating fires destroyed most of the old French Colonial architecture. At the time, New Orleans was under Spanish rule, so much of what you'll see—from wrought-iron balconies to common-wall brick houses— reflects that period.

There's so much to do and see in the Quarter that just one walking tour wouldn't do it justice. Therefore, we offer three separate walks: this one, along with the Back of the Quarter (Walk 5) and French Market/Riverfront (Walk 6).

● **Begin at North Peters and Iberville Streets. Walk four blocks down Iberville. In the fourth block, you'll pass two classic seafood eateries: Acme Oyster House to your left and Felix's to your right. Both places have bars where you can take in the art of oyster shucking. Also on this block are the higher-end Dickie Brennan's Steakhouse and Bourbon House, both run by restaurateur Dickie Brennan, who with other members of the Brennan family owns some of the city's top restaurants.**

- Turn right on Bourbon and brace yourself for the adult-themed playground that lies ahead. Ironically, one of the city's most critically acclaimed restaurants, the legendary Galatoire's, is among the first places you'll pass. Galatoire's dates back to 1905, when Jean Galatoire brought his culinary talents to New Orleans from the village of Pardies, France. Known for its French Creole cooking, Galatoire's boasts such dishes as crabmeat Sardou, chicken Clemenceau, oysters Rockefeller, and shrimp rémoulade. Eating at Galatoire's is the ultimate fine-dining experience, with tuxedoed waiters tending to your every need. If you're a regular, you likely have your own waiter. Although reservations are taken for the second floor, waiting in line for the more festive first floor—especially on Fridays—is the way to have a true Galatoire's experience.

- Continue down Bourbon, where you'll pass strip joints, T-shirt shops, daiquiri shops, and the like. At the end of the block is Jean Lafitte's Old Absinthe House, which opened its doors in 1807. Legend has it that the pirate Jean Lafitte and Andrew Jackson met on the second floor to plan the victory of the Battle of New Orleans. Over the years, the tavern has hosted such celebrities as Frank Sinatra, Mark Twain, and Liza Minnelli. Its interior features antique chandeliers and the jerseys of football legends hanging from the exposed cypress beams.

- In the next block, the Royal Sonesta Hotel is to the right. The Sonesta has long been one of the Crescent City's finest hotels. It's home to Restaurant R'evolution, the latest restaurant of chef John Folse, and Irvin Mayfield's Jazz Playhouse, the jazz club of Grammy Award–winning trumpeter and bandleader Irvin Mayfield. One of the city's musical treasures, Mayfield is an amazing talent who also teaches, composes, and travels the world spreading the gospel of New Orleans jazz. He and his New Orleans Jazz Orchestra perform at the club on Wednesday nights in a show billed as Irvin Mayfield's NOJO Jam; other regulars include the James Rivers Movement, Glen David Andrews, and Shannon Powell. One of the most famous traditions associated with the Sonesta occurs every Mardi Gras, when those lucky enough to book balcony rooms arm themselves with beads to toss to the raucous revelers below. The celebrating begins the Friday before Mardi Gras (Fat Tuesday) with the annual "Greasing of the Poles," a Sonesta-sponsored event in which celebrity greasers spread petroleum jelly on the hotel's supporting poles to prevent partiers from climbing up to the balcony.

● Over the next few blocks you'll pass several more bars and lounges, among them Rick's Cabaret, one of Bourbon Street's fancier strip clubs; the Famous Door, where pianist, actor, and *American Idol* judge Harry Connick Jr. played his first gig at 13 years old; and the Chris Owens Club, a burlesque joint whose ageless namesake is a French Quarter nightlife legend.

The Four Points by Sheraton French Quarter, at 541 Bourbon, occupies the one-time site of the legendary French Opera House, which served as the center of the city's social and cultural life, especially among the Creoles. The Opera House opened in 1859, and New Orleans quickly became known as "The Opera Capital of North America." It remained that way until 1919, when a fire destroyed the building.

At the corner of Bourbon and Toulouse Streets is Tropical Isle, known for a drink called the Hand Grenade, a melon-flavored concoction that, with its mixture of "liqueurs and other secret ingredients," is billed as "New Orleans's most powerful drink." Farther down the block, to the left, is Channing Tatum's Saints and Sinners, the bordello-themed restaurant and bar that Tatum, a regular visitor to New Orleans, opened with a business partner in 2012.

● From Toulouse, walk one block to St. Peter Street and turn right. On this block, you'll pass two of the city's most beloved landmarks: Preservation Hall and Pat O'Brien's. Preservation Hall opened in 1961 to honor traditional New Orleans jazz. Nightly performances feature bands made up of such musicians as Greg Stafford, Charlie Gabriel, and Ernie Elly. All ages are welcome, so if you have children in tow, bring them along for this one-of-a-kind learning experience.

Pat O'Brien's, or Pat O's for short, is a playground within itself, an entertainment mecca since 1933, when, at the end of Prohibition, Pat O'Brien converted his speak-easy to a legal drinking establishment. Pat O's features several bars, among them a patio bar and a piano bar, where dueling entertainers lead sing-alongs from two copper-topped baby grand pianos. The signature drink is the Hurricane, a rum-based libation served in a 26-ounce souvenir glass.

● Walk one block to Royal Street and turn right. Royal is the antithesis of Bourbon: a ritzy shopping stretch lined with antiques shops, art galleries, jewelry stores, and boutiques. Among them are M. S. Rau Antiques, Ida Manheim Antiques, Sutton Gallery, and Vincent Mann Gallery.

At 533 Royal, between St. Louis and Toulouse Streets, is the Historic New Orleans Collection, a museum and research center dedicated to the study and preservation of the history and culture of New Orleans and the Gulf South region. The museum's holdings include more than 35,000 library items; more than 2 miles of documents and manuscripts; and about 350,000 photographs, prints, drawings, paintings, and other artifacts. The updated and interactive Louisiana History Galleries comprises 13 galleries tracing Louisiana's fascinating past. The latest additions to the permanent display are exhibits on Hurricane Katrina and the 2010 BP oil spill.

● Walk one block to 400 Royal. The stunning Beaux Arts structure to the left is the home of the Louisiana Supreme Court. The state's highest court moved into the building in 1910, where it remained for nearly 50 years. After the court moved to the more contemporary Central Business District, the building fell into disrepair, but it saw new life in 2004 when, after a major renovation, the Supreme Court returned to its Royal Street address.

Across the street, at 417 Royal, is Brennan's, the old-line restaurant renowned for its sumptuous breakfasts, world-famous bananas Foster, and romantic courtyard. To the dismay of foodies everywhere, Brennan's shut down in the summer of 2013 after its owners declared bankruptcy, but a cousin, New Orleans restaurateur Ralph Brennan, came to the rescue: He purchased the property at auction, bought back the Brennan's name, and reopened the French Quarter institution in November 2014. Meanwhile, Brennan's former owners were planning to open a new eatery, Ted Brennan's Decatur, on nearby Decatur Street in 2015.

In the next block, at 334 Royal St., is the headquarters of the New Orleans Police Department's Eighth District. Erected in 1826 as the Old Bank of Louisiana, the building served as Louisiana's state capitol from 1868 to 1869, and later the Royal Street Auction Exchange and the Mortgage and Conveyance Office. This block of Royal also contains lots of fun shops, including Vintage 329, which specializes in autographed memorabilia, rare books, and other historical items.

If you need a break—or even if you don't—stop in at the venerable Hotel Monteleone (214 Royal St.), which boasts live entertainment and one of the most popular hotel bars in New Orleans. The Carousel Bar & Lounge features a 25-seat revolving bar with a carousel top, antiqued mirrors, and hand-painted chairs. The lounge, with its circular glass chandeliers and expansive windows along Royal Street, is equally inviting.

● Turn left on Iberville Street, walk one block to Chartres Street, and turn left. Like Royal, Chartres offers a lot in the way of shopping, but it also has much to offer in the way of eating. Over the last few years, Chartres has become something of a culinary corridor, with several new restaurants—SoBou, Doris Metropolitan, Kingfish, Sylvain, Tableau, and a French Quarter outpost of Carrollton's Camellia Grill—joining K-Paul's Louisiana Kitchen and Pierre Maspero's in the five blocks between Iberville and St. Peters Streets.

Of course, you may just opt for the Napoleon House (500 Chartres St.), which has been serving up its famous Pimm's Cups and muffulettas since 1914. The Napoleon House—one of the best bars in America, according to *Esquire* magazine—is housed in a 200-year-old building that belonged to Nicolas Girod, mayor of New Orleans from 1812 to 1815. Girod offered his residence to Napoleon Bonaparte in 1821 as a refuge during his exile; alas, Napoleon died before he could make it to New Orleans.

A few doors down from the Napoleon House is the Pharmacy Museum (514 Chartres St.), the one-time apothecary shop of Louis Joseph Dufilho Jr., who in the early 19th century became America's first licensed pharmacist. On display are old patent medicines, books, and pharmaceutical equipment dating back as far as the early 1800s, as well as surgical instruments used in the Civil War. Other exhibits include a re-created 19th-century physician's study and a spectacle collection ▶

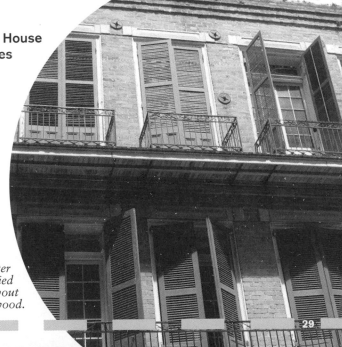

For many New Orleanians, the French Quarter is home. This is an example of a balconied apartment building that can be found throughout the neighborhood.

illustrating the historical development of eyewear and other antique vision aids from around the world.

● Continue walking to the corner of Chartres and St. Peter Streets. To your left is Le Petit Théâtre du Vieux Carré, one of the oldest community theaters in the country. Originally organized in 1916 as the New Orleans Chapter of the Drama League of America, the company began performing in this space in 1922. In 2012 and 2013, the theater underwent a multimillion-dollar renovation that added Tableau, a Dickie Brennan restaurant specializing in Louisiana Creole fare.

● Continue walking on Chartres straight into Jackson Square, the highlight of which is the triple-spired St. Louis Cathedral, the oldest cathedral in North America and easily the city's most recognizable landmark. The church features a Rococo-style gilded altar along with magnificent stained-glass windows and paintings. In the rear of the cathedral is the St. Anthony Garden, where a statue of Jesus stands with arms upraised. Stop in for Mass or a tour; the cathedral is open daily after the 7:30 a.m. Mass until 4 p.m., and self-guided tours are available for a $1 donation.

The cathedral is flanked by the Cabildo and the Presbytère, two of several museums under the Louisiana State Museum umbrella. Facing the cathedral, the Cabildo is to your left. Built in the late 18th century, the Cabildo served as the seat of government in New Orleans during the Spanish Colonial period and is where the Louisiana Purchase—which nearly doubled the size of the United States—was signed in 1803. To your right is the Presbytère, a one-time courthouse that now houses an exquisite collection of Mardi Gras artifacts and memorabilia. Through an interactive exhibit titled "Mardi Gras: It's Carnival Time in Louisiana," visitors can learn the history of Mardi Gras, from its 19th-century beginnings to the modern-day celebration that attracts millions of tourists every year.

Take your time strolling around the square and enjoy the vibrancy of the artists, musicians, and other street performers at work. The redbrick buildings on either side of the square are the Lower and Upper Pontalba Buildings, the oldest apartments in the United States. The apartments take up the top three stories, while shops and restaurants occupy the first. One of the best is Stanley, at the corner of St. Ann and Chartres, a casual eatery known for its all-day breakfast fare. Another restaurant worth checking out is Muriel's Jackson Square, just across St. Ann from Stanley. Muriel's serves contemporary Creole fare and boasts one of the best dining balconies in town.

If you have a few extra minutes to spare, walk through the square, named in honor of General Andrew Jackson, the hero of the Battle of New Orleans. Known in the 18th century as the Place d'Armes, the historic park is a popular site for television broadcasts and music festivals, including the French Quarter Festival and Caroling in the Square.

- Continue walking around the square along Decatur Street, across from Café Du Monde, the famous coffee-and-beignets stand. This block of Decatur is an assembly spot for horse-drawn-carriage tours.

- Walk to St. Peter Street, turn right, and head one more block back to Chartres Street. The tour ends here, but be sure to check out the Back of the Quarter and the French Market/Riverfront area, each covered in the next two walks.

POINTS OF INTEREST

Acme Oyster House acmeoyster.com, 724 Iberville St., 504-522-5973

Dickie Brennan's Steakhouse dickiebrennanssteakhouse.com, 716 Iberville St., 504-522-2467

Felix's Restaurant and Oyster Bar felixs.com, 739 Iberville St., 504-522-4440

Bourbon House bourbonhouse.com, 144 Bourbon St., 504-522-0111

Galatoire's galatoires.com, 209 Bourbon St., 504-525-2021

Jean Lafitte's Old Absinthe House ruebourbon.com/oldabsinthehouse, 240 Bourbon St., 504-523-3181

Royal Sonesta Hotel New Orleans sonesta.com/royalneworleans, 300 Bourbon St., 504-586-0300

Restaurant R'evolution revolutionnola.com, 777 Bienville St., 504-553-2277

Irvin Mayfield's Jazz Playhouse irvinmayfield.com, 300 Bourbon St., 504-553-2299

Famous Door 339 Bourbon St., 504-598-4334

Chris Owens Club chrisowensclub.net, 500 Bourbon St., 504-523-6400

Tropical Isle tropicalisle.com, 600 Bourbon St., 504-529-1702

Saints and Sinners saintsandsinnersnola.com, 627 Bourbon St., 504-528-9307

Preservation Hall preservationhall.com, 726 St. Peter St., 504-522-2841

Pat O'Brien's patobriens.com, 718 St. Peter St., 504-525-4823

Historic New Orleans Collection hnoc.org, 522 Royal St., 504-523-4662

Louisiana Supreme Court lasc.org, 400 Royal St., 504-310-2300

Brennan's brennansneworleans.com, 417 Royal St., 504-525-9711

New Orleans Police Department, Eighth District nola.gov/nopd, 334 Royal St., 504-658-6080

Vintage 329 vintage329.com, 329 Royal St., 504-525-2262

Carousel Bar & Lounge, Hotel Monteleone hotelmonteleone.com, 214 Royal St., 504-523-3341

SoBou sobounola.com, 310 Chartres St., 504-552-4095

Kingfish cocktailbarneworleans.com, 337 Chartres St., 504-598-5005

K-Paul's Louisiana Kitchen chefpaul.com/kpaul, 416 Chartres St., 504-596-2530

Napoleon House napoleonhouse.com, 500 Chartres St., 504-524-9752

Pharmacy Museum pharmacymuseum.org, 514 Chartres St., 504-565-8027

Doris Metropolitan dorismetropolitan.com, 620 Chartres St., 504-267-3500

Sylvain sylvainnola.com, 625 Chartres St., 504-265-8123

Le Petit Théâtre du Vieux Carré lepetittheatre.com, 616 St. Peter St., 504-522-2081

Tableau tableaufrenchquarter.com, 616 St. Peter St., 504-934-3463

The Cabildo crt.state.la.us/louisiana-state-museum, 701 Chartres St., 504-568-6968

St. Louis Cathedral stlouiscathedral.org, Jackson Square, 504-525-9585

The Presbytère crt.state.la.us/louisiana-state-museum, 751 Chartres St., 504-568-6968

Jackson Square nola.gov/parks-and-parkways/parks-squares/jackson-square, bounded by St. Ann, St. Peter, Decatur, and Chartres Streets; 504-658-3200

Stanley stanleyrestaurant.com, 547 St. Ann St., 504-587-0093

Muriel's Jackson Square muriels.com, 801 Chartres St., 504-568-1885

route summary

1. Begin walk at Iberville and North Peters Street.
2. Walk four blocks to Bourbon Street and turn right.
3. Walk five blocks to St. Peter Street and turn right.
4. Walk one block to Royal Street and turn right.
5. Walk five blocks to Iberville and turn left.
6. Walk one block to Chartres Street and turn left.
7. Walk five blocks to St. Peter at Jackson Square.
8. Walk around the square back to Chartres Street.

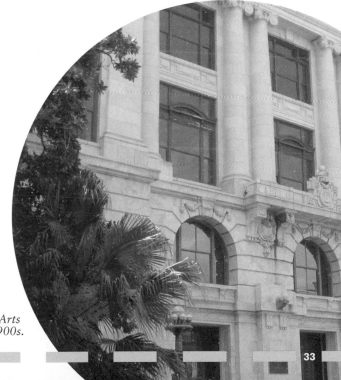

The Louisiana Supreme Court Building is a Beaux Arts structure that dates back to the early 1900s.

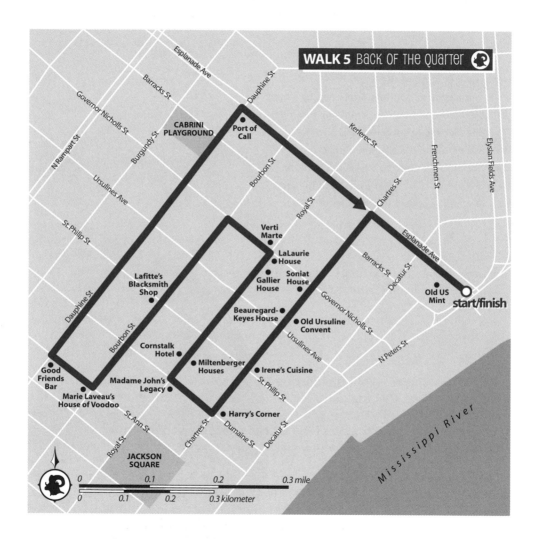

Esplanade Ave

Barracks St

Governor Nicholls St

Burgundy St

N Rampart St

Ursulines Ave

St Philip St

Dauphine St

CABRINI PLAYGROUND

Port of Call

Dauphine St

Bourbon St

Royal St

Kerlerec St

Frenchmen St

Elysian Fields Ave

Chartres St

Esplanade Ave

Verti Marte

LaLaurie House

Gallier House

Soniat House

Barracks St

Decatur St

Old US Mint

start/finish

Lafitte's Blacksmith Shop

Beauregard-Keyes House

Old Ursuline Convent

Governor Nicholls St

Bourbon St

Cornstalk Hotel

Ursulines Ave

N Peters St

Good Friends Bar

Miltenberger Houses

Irene's Cuisine

Madame John's Legacy

Marie Laveau's House of Voodoo

St Ann St

St Philip St

Harry's Corner

Chartres St

Dumaine St

Decatur St

Royal St

JACKSON SQUARE

Mississippi River

| 0 | 0.1 | 0.2 | 0.3 mile |

| 0 | 0.1 | 0.2 | 0.3 kilometer |

5 Back of the Quarter: Spooky Stroll

BOUNDARIES: **Esplanade Ave., Chartres St., Dumaine St., Dauphine St.**
DISTANCE: **1.73 miles**
PARKING: **Limited street parking**
PUBLIC TRANSIT: **RTA Bus #5 (Marigny-Bywater), Riverfront Streetcar**

The French Quarter isn't all about Bourbon Street. In fact, the lower part of the Quarter, between Esplanade Avenue and St. Ann Street, is a mostly residential neighborhood where homes range from restored Creole cottages to French Colonial town houses sporting exquisite wrought-iron balconies. It's relatively quiet, but no less fascinating or historic than its more popular counterpart upriver.

Many of the homes in the Lower French Quarter have been converted to museums, giving visitors an up-close view of 18th- and 19th-century lifestyles; among the more notable examples are the Beauregard-Keyes House and the Gallier House. Some of the city's allegedly haunted houses—like the legendary LaLaurie House—can be found here as well. Even the hotels and inns, such as the Soniat House and the Cornstalk Hotel, have historic significance.

Of course, no New Orleans neighborhood is complete without a culinary component, and two of the best are Irene's Cuisine and Café Amelie, not to mention Verti Marte for po'boys. For libations, Harry's Corner and Lafitte's Blacksmith Shop are among the classics.

● **Begin at the Old US Mint (Esplanade Avenue at North Peters Street),** one of several museums that make up the Louisiana State Museum system. Built in 1835, the Greek Revival building served as a mint for both the Union and the Confederacy. Today, it's home to exhibits on New Orleans jazz, Newcomb pottery, and the Mississippi River, as well as a jazz-performance series called Music at the Mint.

● **Walk two blocks to Chartres Street and turn left.** At 1133 Chartres is the Soniat House, built in the 1820s by Joseph Soniat Dufossat, a French sugar-plantation owner. Now a boutique hotel, the property consists of three town houses with 31 guest rooms furnished and decorated with French and English antiques. It has won many accolades, among them being named one of the top 20 hotels in the world by Fodor's.

- Continue down Chartres. At the end of the block is the Beauregard-Keyes House, a raised center-hall house built in 1826 by architect François Correjolles for auctioneer Joseph LeCarpentier. The house had a number of notable residents over the years, including 19th-century chess master Paul Morphy and Confederate general P. G. T. Beauregard, who rented it from 1866 to 1868 after the Civil War. Novelist Frances Parkinson Keyes, who wrote such historical fiction as *Madame Castel's Lodger* and *Blue Camellia,* lived here from 1945 until her death in 1970. Keyes, with the help of architect Sam Wilson, restored the house and established the Keyes Foundation, which maintains it to this day. The house reflects the years that Beauregard lived there and features furniture and art owned by the general and his family, along with Keyes's writing studio and her extensive collections of dolls and porcelain.

  Across the street is the Old Ursuline Convent, the oldest building in the Mississippi Valley, having been designed and constructed over an eight-year period from 1745 to 1753. The building has served several purposes over the centuries, from convent and school to archbishop's residence and central office of the Archdiocese of New Orleans. It is now the home of the Catholic Cultural Heritage Center.

- Continue down Chartres to St. Philip Street. At the corner to your right is Irene's Cuisine, a French Quarter institution with a great menu of Creole-Italian fare like soft-shell-crab linguini and seafood cioppino. Irene's is so good, and so much fun, that patrons don't seem to mind the inevitable long wait for a table, even with reservations—time flies when you're spending it drinking wine at the cozy little piano bar. In the next block, at the corner of Chartres and Dumaine, is Harry's Corner, treasured by those looking for a French Quarter bar experience away from the craziness of Bourbon Street.

- Walk one more block to Dumaine Street and turn right. At 632 Dumaine is Madame John's Legacy, a complex of 18th-century Louisiana Creole buildings that escaped the Great New Orleans Fire of 1794. Designed in the French West Indies style, it encompasses three buildings: the main house, which is open to the public; the kitchen; and the two-story gentlemen's guest quarters.

- Walk to the end of the block and turn right on Royal Street. At 900, 906, and 910 Royal are the Miltenberger Houses, a row of three town houses built in the 1830s by Marie Miltenberger, a widow whose husband, Dr. Christian Miltenberger, had been renowned for his work with yellow fever patients. The houses, with their cast-iron galleries and floor-to-ceiling windows, are among the most photographed in the Quarter. Next door, at 912 Royal, is Café Amelie, a French restaurant with what *Times-Picayune* restaurant critic Brett Anderson calls "one of the city's most romantic outdoor settings."

Across the street at 915 Royal St. is the Cornstalk Hotel, famous for its cast-iron fence depicting ears of corn intertwined with morning glories. The hotel was built as a residence for Judge François Xavier Martin, chief justice of the Louisiana Supreme Court, who lived there from 1816 to 1826. Dr. Joseph Secondo Biamenti bought the mansion in 1834, converted it to a hotel, and added its famous fence. Prominent guests include Bill and Hillary Clinton, Elvis Presley, and Harriet Beecher Stowe, who used nearby slave quarters as her inspiration for *Uncle Tom's Cabin.*

● Walk two blocks to 1132 Royal St., the residence of noted architect James Gallier and his family during the mid-19th century. The Gallier House, which is open to the public, tells the story of those who lived and worked on the property. In addition to the home itself, the tour ($12 adults, $10 seniors and kids) includes the gardens, carriageway, and restored slave quarters. The house is especially fun to visit in December, when it's embellished in holiday dress.

● Just down the block, at 1140 Royal St., is the LaLaurie House—also known simply as "The Haunted House"—which, along with its evil owner, was featured in the FX series *American Horror Story: Coven.* Madame Delphine LaLaurie, a wealthy socialite, bought the Creole mansion in 1831, and incredible stories of wild parties and servant abuse soon followed. When a fire broke out in 1834, neighbors broke in through a locked door and found seven slaves chained and starving. As outraged citizens protested outside, a carriage sped into the crowd and away from the premises; in the carriage were Madame LaLaurie and her family, who escaped to Paris, never to return. Legend has it that the spirits of the slaves still inhabit the mansion, making it a favorite stop on haunted-history tours.

● Turn left on Governor Nicholls Street. At the corner of Governor Nicholls and Royal is the Verti Marte, a beloved French Quarter institution known for its All That Jazz po'boy (sautéed shrimp, turkey, ham, mushrooms, Swiss and American cheeses, and a special "Wow Sauce"). The place is open 24 hours a day, seven days a week, making it wildly popular with locals.

- Walk one block to Bourbon Street and turn left. Walk two blocks to Lafitte's Blacksmith Shop (941 Bourbon St.), a tavern that was built between 1722 and 1732 and is considered one of the oldest structures used as a bar in the United States. According to Lafitte's website, the property is believed to have been used by pirates Jean and Pierre Lafitte as a New Orleans base for their smuggling operation.

- Walk two blocks to 739 Bourbon St., home of Marie Laveau's House of Voodoo. Named for the city's most famous voodoo queen, this fun souvenir shop sells everything from tribal masks and statues to voodoo dolls and spell kits. And if you want to have your palm read or your fortune told, you're at the right place.

- Head right on St. Ann Street (left if you're leaving the House of Voodoo), walk one block to Dauphine Street, then turn right and take Dauphine five blocks to Esplanade Avenue. At the corner of St. Ann and Dauphine, on your left, you'll pass Good Friends, one of the city's most popular gay bars. Farther up Dauphine, you'll also pass Cabrini Playground on your right, between Governor Nicholls and Barracks Streets. Yes, there is an actual playground in the French Quarter (along with two schools), because families with young children really do live here.

- Turn right on Esplanade Avenue. As you round the corner, don't be surprised to see a crowd of people standing in front of 838 Esplanade—this is Port of Call, which, even with the proliferation of burger restaurants across town, is considered one of the city's best.

- Walk five blocks back to your starting point at the Old US Mint.

POINTS OF INTEREST

Old US Mint crt.state.la.us, 400 Esplanade Ave., 504-568-2022

Soniat House soniathouse.com, 1133 Chartres St., 504-522-0570

Beauregard-Keyes House bkhouse.org, 1113 Chartres St., 504-523-7257

Old Ursuline Convent oldursulineconvent.org, 1100 Chartres St., 504-529-3040

Irene's Cuisine 539 St. Philip St., 504-529-8811

Harry's Corner 900 Chartres St., 504-524-1107

Madame John's Legacy crt.state.la.us/louisiana-state-museum, 632 Dumaine St., 504-568-6968

Miltenberger Houses 900, 906, and 910 Royal St.

Café Amelie cafeamelie.com, 912 Royal St., 504-412-8965

Cornstalk Hotel cornstalkhotel.com, 915 Royal St., 504-523-1515

Gallier House hgghh.org, 1132 Royal St., 504-525-5661

LaLaurie House 1140 Royal St.

Verti Marte 1201 Royal St., 504-525-4767

Lafitte's Blacksmith Shop lafittesblacksmithshop.com, 941 Bourbon St., 504-593-9761

Marie Laveau's House of Voodoo voodooneworleans.com, 739 Bourbon St., 504-581-3751

Good Friends Bar goodfriendsbar.com, 740 Dauphine St., 504-566-7191

Cabrini Playground Dauphine Street between Governor Nicholls and Barracks Streets

Port of Call portofcallnola.com, 838 Esplanade Ave., 504-523-0120

route summary

1. Begin on Esplanade Avenue at North Peters Street.
2. Walk two blocks to Chartres Street.
3. Turn left and walk five blocks to Dumaine Street.
4. Turn right and walk one block to Royal Street.
5. Turn right and walk three blocks to Governor Nicholls Street.
6. Turn left and walk one block to Bourbon Street.
7. Turn left and walk four blocks to St. Ann Street.
8. Turn right and walk one block to Dauphine Street.
9. Turn right and walk five blocks to Esplanade Avenue.
10. Turn right and walk five blocks to North Peters Street.

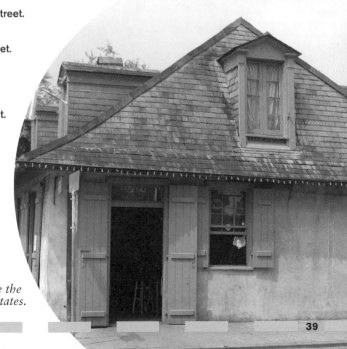

Lafitte's Blacksmith Shop is believed to be the oldest structure used as a bar in the United States.

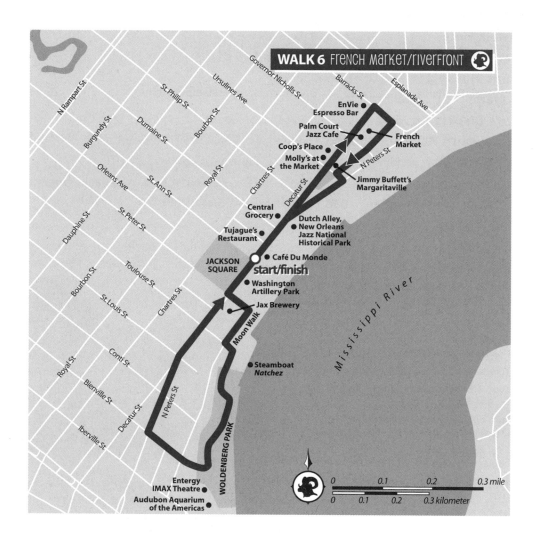

Governor Nicholls St

Barracks St

Esplanade Ave

Ursulines Ave

N Rampart St

St Philip St

Burgundy St

Dumaine St

Bourbon St

Orleans Ave

St Ann St

Royal St

Dauphine St

St Peter St

Chartres St

Decatur St

EnVie
Espresso Bar

Palm Court
Jazz Cafe

French
Market

Coop's Place

N Peters St

Molly's at
the Market

Jimmy Buffett's
Margaritaville

Central
Grocery

Dutch Alley,
New Orleans
Jazz National
Historical Park

Tujague's
Restaurant

**JACKSON
SQUARE**

Café Du Monde

start/finish

Washington
Artillery Park

Bourbon St

Toulouse St

St Louis St

Chartres St

Jax Brewery

Moon Walk

Steamboat
Natchez

Mississippi River

Royal St

Conti St

Bienville St

N Peters St

Decatur St

Iberville St

WOLDENBERG PARK

Entergy
IMAX Theatre

Audubon Aquarium
of the Americas

0   0.1   0.2   0.3 mile

0   0.1   0.2   0.3 kilometer

6 French Market/Riverfront: Family Fun in the Quarter

BOUNDARIES: Bienville St., Decatur St., Barracks St., Mississippi River
DISTANCE: 1.62 miles
PARKING: Several parking lots along Decatur
PUBLIC TRANSIT: Riverfront Streetcar, RTA Buses #5 (Marigny-Bywater) and #55 (Elysian Fields)

The Riverfront area between Canal Street and Esplanade Avenue may be part of the French Quarter, but it's also a world within itself: a vibrant mix of attractions that includes the lively French Market, a riverfront promenade, and a linear park with lush pathways and stunning sculptures.

Founded in 1791, the French Market is the oldest public market in the United States. Stretching six blocks from Barracks Street to St. Ann Street, it was established as a Native American trading post and at one time was the only legal place in the city to buy meat. Its latest incarnation is that of a culinary corridor complete with countertop dining, a cooking demonstration stage, and live musical performances.

Other focal points of the area include the Moon Walk, a riverfront walkway with spectacular views; Woldenberg Park, among the treasures of the Audubon Nature Institute; and the world-famous Café Du Monde, which has been serving café au lait and sugar-laden beignets since 1862.

Annual festivals add to the frivolity of the Riverfront, including the French Quarter Festival, the Creole Tomato Festival, the Bastille Day Fête, and the Mighty Mississippi River Festival. If you have kids in tow, bring them along—the French Quarter, at least this part of it, truly is a family destination.

● Begin your walk in front of River's Edge, a restaurant at the corner of Decatur and St. Ann Streets in Jackson Square. Walk upriver, away from the square, to the corner of Madison Avenue, home of Tujague's, the Crescent City's second oldest restaurant. It's known as much for its bar as it is for its Creole fare: The cypress stand-up bar and ornate French mirror behind it have been part of this institution since it opened in 1856.

AUDUBON AQUARIUM OF THE AMERICAS

From the moment you walk through the underwater tunnel at the Audubon Aquarium of the Americas, you know you've arrived at a special place. Part of the Aquarium's Caribbean Reef Exhibit, the glass-enclosed tunnel is surrounded by a 132,000-gallon tank where exotic creatures such as angelfish, cownose rays, and moray eels swim about to the delight of visitors.

The tunnel is one of the Aquarium's trademark features, but it's just the beginning of a fascinating journey through the waters of the Americas, from the Amazon to the Caribbean.

The interactive Geaux Fish! Exhibit showcases Louisiana's fishing industry and invites you to cast a virtual reel, identify local species, visit a seafood market, and board a fishing boat. Parakeet Pointe is an 800-square-foot outdoor area where you can meander among hundreds of vibrant parakeets and, for a minimal charge, buy seed sticks and feed the birds.

You can even experience the Amazon Orinoco rainforest by climbing into the Amazon "tree-top loop" and marveling at such exotic species of fish as payara piranhas, pacu fish, and freshwater stingrays. One of the aquarium's most popular sites is the Penguin Exhibit, featuring a colony of penguins from South America and Africa.

Be sure to pick up a schedule of feedings, chats, and other daily events at the information booth. And if time allows, pair your visit to the Aquarium with tickets to the Entergy IMAX Theatre just next door, where you can choose from an array of award-winning nature films. The theater's five-and-a-half-story screen—the largest IMAX screen in the Gulf South—makes for an unmatched viewing experience.

● Walk one block to Central Grocery, a small Italian market where the famous muffuletta was invented by founder Salvatore Lupo, a Sicilian immigrant, back in 1906. The muffuletta is a sandwich made with round Italian bread and stuffed with cold cuts, cheese, and olive salad. In addition to Italian delicacies, the market sells a variety of French, Spanish, Greek, and Creole specialty foods. Stop in, if only to take a whiff.

● Continue walking down Decatur, where you'll pass numerous souvenir and T-shirt shops, including one called the Jazz Funeral. In the block between Ursulines Avenue and Governor Nicholls Street, you'll pass Molly's at the Market, the city's unofficial media bar, and Coop's Place, a great place to grab some grub after a night at Molly's. Cane & Table is known for its rum-inspired drinks and island-themed fare. Across the street is Jimmy Buffett's Margaritaville, which serves up an island-inspired menu and live music from 3 p.m. at the eatery's Storyville Tavern.

● In the next block, to your right, is the Palm Court Jazz Cafe, where you can listen to traditional New Orleans jazz while dining on such Louisiana fare as red beans and rice, crawfish pie, and Creole gumbo. Nina Buck and her late husband, jazz musician George Buck, opened Palm Court in 1989 in a fully restored early-19th-century building. In addition to the Palm Court Jazz Band, regular performers include Clive Wilson's New Orleans Serenaders; the Crescent City Joymakers; and musicians Mark Braud and Lars Edegran. Trumpeter Lionel Ferbos, the Palm Court Jazz Band's longtime frontman, was considered New Orleans's oldest working musician. (Ferbos, who died in July 2014 at age 103, performed regularly until 2013.) Need a break? Check out EnVie Espresso Bar & Café for its impressive menu of coffee drinks and pastries.

● Walk to Barracks Street, turn right, and enter the back side of the French Market. The market has undergone numerous changes since it opened in 1791, but one thing that hasn't changed is its status as a cultural and commercial icon. This six-block stretch includes a vibrant Flea Market, where vendors sell jewelry, artwork, candles, and other merchandise 365 days a year. The Flea Market leads to the Farmers Market, which has a variety of food stands along with fresh produce, seafood, and baked goods. Eateries include Alberto's Cheese & Wine Bistro; Continental Provisions, J's Seafood Dock; and Meals From The Heart Café, which serves vegetarian, vegan, and gluten-free fare. The guys shucking oysters are a show in themselves.

● Continue walking through the Farmers Market to Ursulines Avenue. Turn left, then turn right at North Peters Street. To your right is Latrobe Park, a lush green space where you can take a break on one of the benches and enjoy the sounds of jazz coming from the nearby Gazebo Café. Dedicated to architect Benjamin Latrobe, the park sits on the site of the city's first waterworks, which Latrobe designed. He died from yellow fever in 1820 as he was working on the project.

- Walk a block to St. Philip Street. To your right is Place de France, a tiny park that houses a golden bronze statue of Joan of Arc atop a horse. The equestrian statue, a gift from France to New Orleans in 1959, is a replica of the 1880 Emmanuel Fremiet statue in the Place des Pyramides in Paris.

- At this point, North Peters turns into Decatur Street. Continue walking past the myriad shops that line the next block. Stop in one of the praline shops along the way. Most are more than happy to let you sample their confections.

- Walk a block to Dumaine Street. To the left is Dutch Alley, a promenade that runs parallel to North Peters. Named for former Mayor Ernest "Dutch" Morial, Dutch Alley is home to an artists' co-op managed and operated by nearly two dozen craftspeople. Original art on display includes jewelry, photography, paintings, pottery, fabric art, and works made from salvaged materials and glass. In the same area is the New Orleans Jazz National Historical Park, which presents jazz performances, lectures, films, and exhibits.

- At the corner of St. Ann and Decatur is the Café Du Monde, known for its café au lait (half coffee, half milk) and beignets, square pieces of dough fried and covered with powdered sugar. This is the original Café Du Monde, which opened in 1862 and continues to operate seven days a week, 24 hours a day (except on Christmas Day).

- From the side of the Café Du Monde, take the stairs up to Washington Artillery Park, a raised plaza that pays homage to the 141st Field Artillery of the Louisiana National Guard, the oldest artillery unit in the United States. The park features a replica of a cannon used in the Civil War. With Jackson Square and St. Louis Cathedral on one side and the Mississippi River on the other side, this is one of the most photographed spots in New Orleans.

- Take the stairs down to the ground level, and cross the parking lot and streetcar tracks to the entrance of the Moon Walk, a riverfront promenade where you can relax on a bench and enjoy the views. The Moon Walk is named for former Mayor Moon Landrieu, under whose leadership the walkway opened in the 1970s.

- Once on the Moon Walk, turn right and continue walking. Among the landmarks that you'll pass are the Jax Brewery, to your right, a shopping mall that once served as the brewhouse for Jax Beer. The four floors of stores, restaurants, bars, and attractions include the Jax Collection, a museum where you can learn the fascinating history of Jax Beer. To your left is the Toulouse Street Wharf, which serves as the entrance for the Steamboat *Natchez,* the last authentic steamboat on the Mississippi. The *Natchez* offers a variety of jazz and dining cruises.

● The Moon Walk leads to Woldenberg Riverfront Park, named for philanthropist Malcolm Woldenberg. The 16-acre park features a jogging path along with artwork and sculptures, including a stunning Holocaust Memorial Exhibit. The park is a backdrop for the French Quarter Festival, the New Orleans Oyster Festival, and the Zulu Lundi Gras Festival, among other big-time events. It is part of the Audubon Nature Institute, which also operates the Aquarium of the Americas (see sidebar) and the Entergy IMAX Theatre, both of which are adjacent to the park. Exit the park via Bienville Street.

● Turn right on North Peters Street and walk two blocks to Toulouse Street. North Peters becomes Decatur Street. Walk four blocks down Decatur back to your starting point.

POINTS OF INTEREST

Tujague's Restaurant tujaguesrestaurant.com, 823 Decatur St., 504-525-8676

Central Grocery 923 Decatur St., 504-523-1620

Jimmy Buffett's Margaritaville margaritavilleneworleans.com, 1104 Decatur St., 504-592-2565

Molly's at the Market mollysatthemarket.net, 1107 Decatur St., 504-525-5169

Coop's Place coopsplace.net, 1109 Decatur St., 504-525-9053

Cane & Table caneandtablenola.com, 1113 Decatur St., 504-581-1112

Palm Court Jazz Cafe palmcourtjazzcafe.com, 1204 Decatur St., 504-525-0200

EnVie Espresso Bar & Cafe nolalovescoffee.com/envie-espresso-bar-cafe, 1241 Decatur St., 504-524-3689

French Market frenchmarket.org, 1235 N. Peters St., 504-596-3420

Dutch Alley Artist's Co-op dutchalleyartistsco-op.com, 912 N. Peters St., 504-412-9220

New Orleans Jazz National Historical Park nps.gov/jazz, 916 N. Peters St., 504-589-4841

Café Du Monde cafedumonde.com, 800 Decatur St., 504-525-4544

Washington Artillery Park frenchmarket.org/venue/washington-artillery-park, 749 Decatur St., 504-596-3420

Jax Brewery jacksonbrewery.com, 600 Decatur St., 504-566-7245

Steamboat *Natchez* steamboatnatchez.com, Toulouse Street Wharf, 504-569-1401

Woldenberg Riverfront Park auduboninstitute.org/visit/aquarium/exhibits-and-attractions /woldenberg-park, 1 Canal St., 504-565-3033

Entergy IMAX Theatre auduboninstitute.org/visit/imax, 1 Canal St., 504-565-3033

Audubon Aquarium of the Americas auduboninstitute.org/visit/aquarium, 1 Canal St., 504-565-3033

route summary

1. Begin walk at St. Ann and Decatur Streets.
2. Walk six blocks to Barracks Street and turn right.
3. Cross Decatur and walk 1½ blocks to back entrance of French Market.
4. Walk two blocks through Flea Market and Farmers Market.
5. Turn left at Ursulines Avenue, then right onto North Peters.
6. Walk one block to St. Philip Street, where North Peters turns into Decatur.
7. Walk down Decatur to Washington Artillery Park (across from Jackson Square).
8. Take stairs from park, and cross parking lot and streetcar tracks to entrance of Moon Walk.
9. Turn right and walk along the Moon Walk to Woldenberg Park.
10. Walk through park toward Aquarium of the Americas.
11. Turn right at Bienville Street.
12. Leave park via Bienville. At North Peters, turn right and walk two blocks to Toulouse, where North Peters turns into Decatur.
13. Walk four blocks on Decatur back to your starting point.

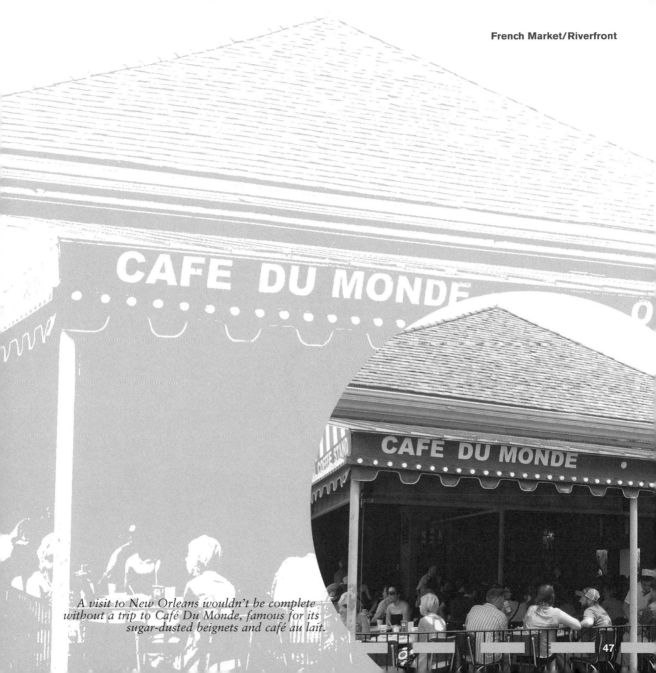

A visit to New Orleans wouldn't be complete without a trip to Café Du Monde, famous for its sugar-dusted beignets and café au lait.

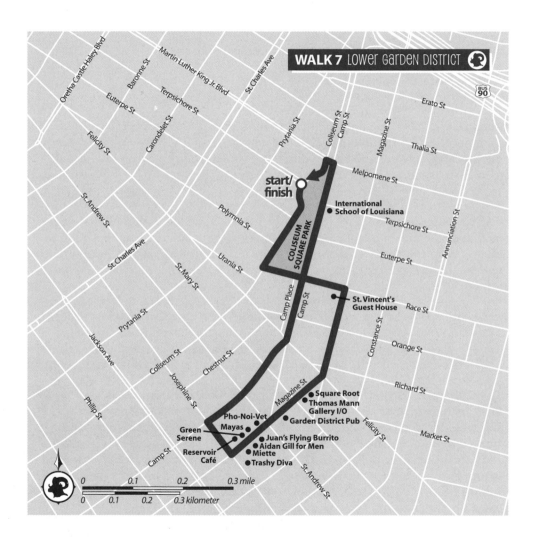

BUS 90

Oretha Castle Haley Blvd

Baronne St

Martin Luther King Jr. Blvd

St. Charles Ave

Terpsichore St

Euterpe St

Carondelet St

Felicity St

Prytania St

Coliseum St

Camp St

Magazine St

Erato St

Thalia St

Melpomene St

St. Andrew St

Polymnia St

start/
finish

**International
School of Louisiana**

Terpsichore St

Annunciation St

St. Charles Ave

St. Mary St

Urania St

COLISEUM
SQUARE PARK

Euterpe St

Prytania St

Camp Place

Camp St

**St. Vincent's
Guest House**

Race St

Constance St

Orange St

Jackson Ave

Coliseum St

Chestnut St

Richard St

Philip St

Josephine St

Magazine St

**Square Root
Thomas Mann
Gallery I/O**

Felicity St

Market St

Pho-Noi-Vet

Mayas

Garden District Pub

**Green
Serene**

Juan's Flying Burrito

Aidan Gill for Men

Miette

**Reservoir
Café**

Trashy Diva

Camp St

St. Andrew St

N

0   0.1   0.2   0.3 mile

0   0.1   0.2   0.3 kilometer

7 Lower Garden District: Preservation Paradise

BOUNDARIES: **Coliseum St., Magazine St., Josephine St., Melpomene St.**
DISTANCE: **1.35 miles**
PARKING: **Free and metered parking**
PUBLIC TRANSIT: **St. Charles Ave. Streetcar**

The Lower Garden District is situated just downriver from the Garden District, but the two neighborhoods are nothing alike. And that's a good thing, because it gives visitors and locals alike a chance to explore yet another area rich in history, beauty, and, in the case of the Lower Garden District, funkiness.

Developed in the early 19th century by architect Barthélemy Lafon, the Lower Garden District boasts elegant mansions that date back to the Civil War, along with a grand square and streets named after the nine muses of Greek mythology. Although the neighborhood saw its share of tough times in the mid-20th century, with many Greek Revival and Italianate mansions falling into decline, preservationists and an active neighborhood association spearheaded its comeback.

Today, the Lower Garden District is a vibrant neighborhood with a funky commercial stretch that includes restaurants, galleries, salons, boutiques, and bars. The association is as active as ever, helping maintain the area's parks and green spaces, working with police and firefighters to enhance safety, and working toward the remediation of blighted properties.

● **Begin at Coliseum and Terpsichore Streets in front of Coliseum Square, a lush neighborhood park with live oaks, walking trails, a fountain, and benches. Facing the park, turn left and walk three blocks to Race Street. To the right, you'll pass some of the neighborhood's most exquisite homes. Among them, at 1741 Coliseum, is a double-gallery Greek Revival house built in 1847 for commission merchant Hugh Wilson. At 1749 Coliseum is the one-time home of Grace King, a Louisiana historian and author who lived there from 1905 to 1932. Built in 1847 by banker Frederick Rodewald, the Greek Revival house has both Ionic and Corinthian columns.**

● Turn left at Race Street and walk three blocks to Magazine Street. Turn right on Magazine in front of St. Vincent's Guest House, which was founded as St. Vincent's Infant Asylum in 1861 by the Daughters of Charity, an order of nuns. (Orphanages were a sad necessity back then because of the thousands of people who were dying from yellow fever.) St. Vincent's later became a home for unwed mothers but shut its doors in the 1970s, largely because of high operating expenses. The building remained empty until Peter Schreiber and Sally Leonard bought it, remodeled it, and opened it as a guest house in 1994.

● Walk three blocks on Magazine to Felicity Street and veer right, continuing on Magazine past such restaurants as Juan's Flying Burrito, Garden District Pub, Mayas Nueva Latino, Pho-Noi-Vet, Reservoir Café, and one of the area's most talked-about restaurants: the acclaimed Square Root. Chef Phillip Lopez offers a tasting menu of 12–15 dishes—kept a surprise until they come to the table—for $150 per person, excluding drinks and tips. No worries if the place isn't in your budget: The second floor is home to Root^2, a no-reservations artisanal charcuterie and cheese studio with a full bar.

This stretch also features some of Magazine's most eclectic shops, among them Thomas Mann Gallery I/O, whose owner, Thomas Mann, is an acclaimed jewelry and functional-art designer. Mann developed what he calls the Techno-Romantic style of design in 1977, combining "industrial aesthetics and materials with evocative themes and romantic imagery." The gallery, which Mann opened in 1988, houses the largest collection of his jewelry, along with home accessories and gifts by dozens of other artists. Other shops include Trashy Diva, a vintage-clothing boutique; Aidan Gill for Men, an upscale men's clothing store; Green Serene, a boutique specializing in sustainable and locally made products; and Miette, a fun jewelry and gift store.

● Turn right on Josephine Street and walk one block to Camp Street. Turn right on Camp and walk five blocks to Coliseum Square. Continue on Camp to Terpsichore. To your right is the International School of Louisiana, a charter school founded in 2000 by a group of parents who wanted a foreign language–based academic program for their children. The school, which has two other campuses in the New Orleans area, was the state's first language-immersion charter school. In 2007, it was named a Charter School of the Year by the Center for Education Reform, the nation's leading education-advocacy organization. The school emphasizes French- and Spanish-language immersion, international awareness, the celebration of diversity, and community responsibility.

● Continue walking around the square to Melpomene Street. Turn left at Melpomene, then left on Coliseum and back to the starting point.

POINTS OF INTEREST

Coliseum Square Park 1700 Coliseum St.

St. Vincent's Guest House stvguesthouse.com, 1507 Magazine St., 504-302-9606

Square Root squarerootnola.com, 1800 Magazine St., 504-309-7800

Thomas Mann Gallery I/O thomasmann.com, 1812 Magazine St., 504-581-2113

Garden District Pub gardendistrictpub.com, 1916 Magazine St., 504-267-3392

Juan's Flying Burrito juansflyingburrito.com, 2018 Magazine St., 504-569-0000

Aidan Gill for Men aidangillformen, 2026 Magazine St., 504-587-9090

Mayas mojitoland.com, 2027 Magazine St., 504-309-3401

Miette iheartmiette.com, 2038 Magazine St., 504-522-2883

Green Serene greenserenenola.com, 2041 Magazine St., 504-252-9861

Reservoir Café reservoircafe.com, 2045 Magazine St., 504-324-5633

Trashy Diva trashydiva.com, 2048 Magazine St., 504-299-8777

International School of Louisiana isl-edu.org, 1400 Camp St., 504-654-1088

route summary

1. Begin walk at Coliseum Street and Terpsichore Street.
2. Facing the Coliseum Square, turn right and walk three blocks to Race Street.
3. Turn left and walk three blocks to Magazine Street.
4. Turn right and walk five blocks to Josephine Street.
5. Turn right and walk one block to Camp Street.
6. Turn right and walk five blocks to Coliseum Square.
7. Continue three blocks on Camp to Melpomene Street.
8. Turn left and walk one block to Coliseum.
9. Turn left and walk one block to the starting point at Coliseum and Terpsichore.

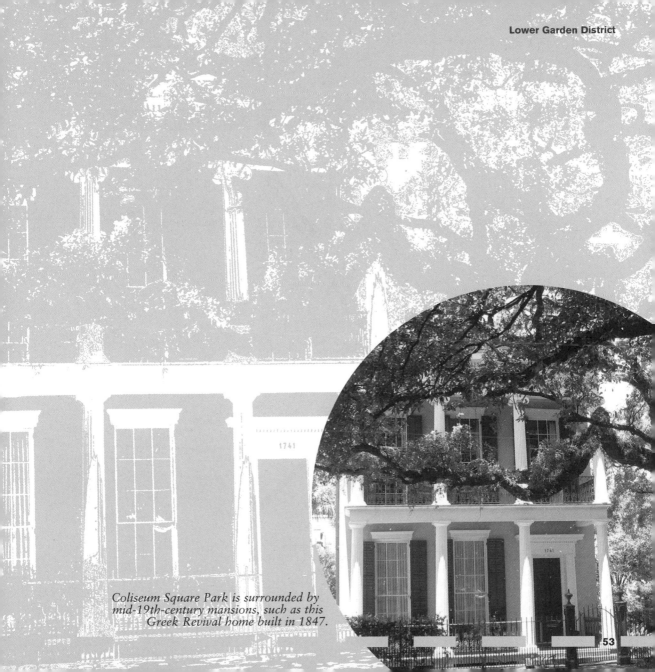

Coliseum Square Park is surrounded by mid-19th-century mansions, such as this Greek Revival home built in 1847.

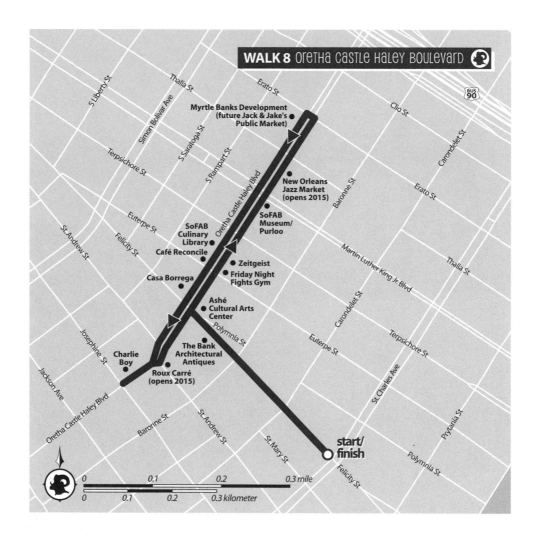

BUS 90

Thalia St

S Liberty St

Simon Bolivar Ave

Terpsichore St

S Saratoga St

S Rampart St

Erato St

Clio St

Carondelet St

Myrtle Banks Development
(future Jack & Jake's
Public Market)

Euterpe St

Felicity St

St Andrew St

New Orleans
Jazz Market
(opens 2015)

Baronne St

Erato St

Oretha Castle Haley Blvd

SoFAB
Museum/
Purloo

SoFAB
Culinary
Library

Café Reconcile

Zeitgeist

Casa Borrega

Friday Night
Fights Gym

Ashé
Cultural Arts
Center

Martin Luther King Jr. Blvd

Thalia St

Carondelet St

Polymnia St

Euterpe St

Terpsichore St

Josephine St

Charlie
Boy

The Bank
Architectural
Antiques

Roux Carré
(opens 2015)

Jackson Ave

St Charles Ave

Pytania St

Oretha Castle Haley Blvd

Baronne St

St Andrew St

St Mary St

start/
finish

Polymnia St

Felicity St

| 0 | | 0.1 | | 0.2 | | 0.3 mile |
| 0 | 0.1 | | 0.2 | | 0.3 kilometer | |

8 Oretha Castle Haley Boulevard: renaissance in the works

BOUNDARIES: **Oretha Castle Haley Blvd., Erato St., Josephine St., St. Charles Ave.**
DISTANCE: **1.39 miles**
PARKING: **Free parking on the street**
PUBLIC TRANSIT: **RTA Buses #15 (Freret) and #91 (Jackson-Esplanade),**
St. Charles Ave. Streetcar

Revival is a theme of many a New Orleans neighborhood, and none may exemplify the concept of comeback more than Oretha Castle Haley Boulevard, one of the main thoroughfares of the historic Central City neighborhood.

A bustling retail strip from the turn of the 20th century through the 1970s, with African American and Jewish merchants running most of the businesses, the street formerly known as Dryades succumbed to disinvestment, poverty, and lack of opportunity. Just blocks away from tony St. Charles Avenue, it became a virtual ghost town, with blighted buildings lining the street and the crime rate continuing to rise.

Fed up with the decline, community activists, civic organizations, and the city of New Orleans embarked on a battle to bring the street affectionately known as O. C. Haley Boulevard— renamed after a beloved civil rights activist in 1989—back to its former glory. Much work remains to be done. But signs of success are everywhere, with restaurants, an independent movie theater, a cultural center, and a gallery among the businesses that have opened shop.

Since 2006, the O. C. Haley Boulevard Merchants & Business Association has sponsored the Central City Festival, an annual all-day celebration that aims to call attention to the street's rebirth. Over the years, some of the city's hottest local musicians, from Kermit Ruffins to Irvin Mayfield, have performed.

● **Begin at St. Charles Avenue and Felicity Street in front of Houston's Restaurant. Facing Felicity, turn right (northwest) and walk three blocks to O. C. Haley Boulevard. Along this stretch of blocks, you'll pass The Muses Apartments, a mixed-income**

café reconcile

If you're looking for flavorful Southern cuisine at an affordable price, look no farther than the corner of Euterpe Street and Oretha Castle Haley Boulevard, home of Café Reconcile.

Not only will you leave with a very satisfied tummy, but you'll have contributed to one of New Orleans's greatest nonprofit success stories.

Café Reconcile opened in 2000, the brainchild of the late Rev. Harry Tompson, who joined with other community members in looking for ways to alleviate the violence, substance abuse, and homelessness that were overtaking the neighborhood. They came up with the idea of a restaurant that would train at-risk youth in the city's thriving hospitality industry.

On any given weekday, the place is packed for lunch. Teens age 16 and older, along with young adults up to age 22, work in all areas of the restaurant, from steward to waitstaff to chef. The service is excellent as is the food, with fried catfish, baked macaroni and cheese, and smothered pork chops among the specialties. Since its beginning, Café Reconcile has seen more than 1,000 of its graduates move on to careers in restaurants, hospitals, and other food-service providers.

The café's partners include some of the city's top chefs and restaurateurs, among them Emeril Lagasse, Ralph Brennan, and John Besh. The Emeril Lagasse Foundation Hospitality Center, a special-events space, occupies the second floor.

housing development built after Hurricane Katrina through a variety of public and private partnerships. The complex gets its name from the surrounding streets, which are named for the nine Muses of Greek mythology.

● Turn right on O. C. Haley. In the first block, at 1712 O. C. Haley, is the Ashé Cultural Arts Center. Housed in what was once Kaufman's Department Store, it opened in the late 1990s. Its mission: to use art and culture to support community development. In addition to staging an array of performing- and visual-arts shows, the center offers movie screenings, health-and-wellness activities, and outreach programs. The Diaspora Boutique sells an abundance of African merchandise from clothing to jewelry.

● Continue walking on O. C. Haley. In the next block, at 1632 O. C. Haley, is the Friday Night Fights Gym, which stages amateur boxing bouts outside Blind Pelican, a nearby bar at St. Charles Avenue and Euterpe Street. The event typically includes musical and dance performances.

At 1618 O. C. Haley is the Zeitgeist Multi-Disciplinary Arts Center, which presents alternative films and other art forms. The center is also home to Church Alley Coffee Bar and the OCH Art Market, which opened in 2010 to help bring foot traffic back to the street. Open the second Saturday of every month, the market invites vendors to sell their crafts, and fresh produce from the Hollygrove Market and Farm is also available.

● Continue walking to 1504 O. C. Haley, home of the Southern Food and Beverage Museum, also known as SoFAB. The museum opened in 2008 at Riverwalk Marketplace downtown but outgrew its space. In late 2014, it reopened in this 30,000-square-foot building, the former Dryades Market. In addition to culinary-themed changing exhibits, the museum houses the Museum of the American Cocktail (hey, it's New Orleans); the Leah Chase Louisiana Gallery (named for the legendary New Orleans chef); and the Gallery of the South: States of Taste, where visitors can explore the cooking cultures of other Southern states. Of course, a museum like this wouldn't be complete without food and drink, so an abundance of space is devoted to a cooking-demo kitchen, along with Purloo, an eatery specializing in regional Southern cuisine.

● In the next block, at the corner of O. C. Haley and Martin Luther King Boulevards, sits the future headquarters of the New Orleans Jazz Market, a project of the New Orleans Jazz Orchestra, which bought the 11,000-square-foot building in 2013. The space, once the home of Gator's department store, will offer music-education classes and performances as well as house a New Orleans jazz archive. The complex will also have a Walk of Fame, which will have as its first inductees trumpeter Irvin Mayfield, singer Dee Dee Bridgewater, and jazz pianist Ellis Marsalis. The project is scheduled for completion in early 2015.

● Walk two blocks to Erato Street, cross O. C. Haley, and turn left to walk on the opposite side of the street. The building at 1307 O. C. Haley is the old Myrtle Banks Elementary School, which as of this writing was being converted to a fresh-food market and an office building. The building opened in 1910 as McDonogh 38 Elementary School but was closed in 2002 because of low enrollment. Six years later, a fire swept through the building, transforming it into blighted eyesore. As part of the neighborhood's revitalization, Alembic Community Development bought and began renovating the property in 2011. Like the New Orleans Jazz Market, this market is set to open in early 2015.

● Walk one block to 1409 O. C. Haley, where you'll be in front of the Harrell Building, a $20 million redevelopment project named for the late Rev. Louis B. Harrell, a long-time resident of Central City and founder of the storefront Living Witness Church of God in Christ in 1981. Harrell was best known for his efforts to improve the quality of life in Central City, starting a clothing-distribution center, a community meal program, a prison ministry, a drug-rehabilitation program, and educational programs aimed at youth. The building houses senior-citizen apartments, office space, and a violence-reduction program called CeaseFire New Orleans. It is also home to the New Orleans Redevelopment Authority, which works with public and private partners to redevelop and revitalize New Orleans neighborhoods like Central City.

● Cross Terpsichore Street. At the corner is Haley's Harvest, one of dozens of community gardens, urban farms, and orchards in underserved New Orleans neighborhoods. In the middle of the block, at 1609 O. C. Haley, is the SoFAB (Southern Food and Beverage) Culinary Library and Archive, which boasts an impressive collection of more than 11,000 volumes of cookbooks; over 5,000 menus; and countless recipes, documents, and other literature about the culinary traditions of the American South. The library is run by the Southern Food and Beverage Museum.

● At the end of the block is the neighborhood's crown jewel: Café Reconcile, a nonprofit restaurant that provides job and life-skills training to at-risk youth (see sidebar).

● A block farther, at 1719 O. C. Haley, is Casa Borrega, which brought authentic Mexican street food and lively Latino entertainment to the neighborhood when it opened in 2012. The restaurant is housed in an 1891 Greek Revival home that had fallen in disrepair when spouses Hugo Montero and Linda Stone purchased it in 2008. In renovating the building, they used as many existing features as possible while adding materials salvaged from buildings in New Orleans, Texas, and Mexico. The menu boasts such dishes as enchiladas de mole, fish tacos, and huevos rancheros, along with more than 100 tequilas and mezcals.

- Walk four blocks to Josephine Street past the headquarters of the Central City Renaissance Alliance, a resident-led community-development organization that envisions a "Central City where the quality of life for everyone is defined by high-quality schools, full employment, an abundance of business and entrepreneurial opportunities, and a healthy and safe environment." At 2043 O. C. Haley is one of the newest additions to the street: Charlie Boy, a high-end men's consignment store.

- Cross O. C. Haley at Josephine. Turn left on O. C. Haley and continue walking. On your right, the Franz Building (2016 O. C. Haley) houses the Good Work Network, a nonprofit that helps start and grow minority- and women-owned businesses; the Trafigura Work and Learn Center, a youth-employment program comprising several youth-run businesses; and the Southeast Louisiana Women's Business Center.

- At the corner of O. C. Haley and St. Andrew Street is the future home of Roux Carré, an outdoor food court and gathering place which, when completed in 2015, will celebrate African American, Caribbean, and Latin American cultures. A project of Good Work Network, the space will feature six food-vendor stalls; a community kitchen; outdoor seating; and staging areas for performances, food demonstrations, and arts markets. Vendors will include chef Linda Green, "The Ya-Ka-Mein Lady," a New Orleans institution known for *ya-ka-mein*—a noodle, meat, and hard-boiled-egg concoction that's popular at local fairs and festivals (and reputed to be a hangover cure).

- Turn right on Felicity Street, past the future restaurant of Chef Adolfo Garcia, whose other establishments include High Hat Cafe and Ancora Pizzeria on Freret Street. Walk three blocks back to the starting point on St. Charles Avenue. Along the way, you'll pass The Bank Architectural Antiques (1824 Felicity), which specializes in antique building materials such as doors, mantels, and period hardware.

POINTS OF INTEREST

Ashé Cultural Arts Center ashecac.org, 1712 Oretha Castle Haley Blvd., 504-569-9070

Friday Night Fights Gym 1630 Oretha Castle Haley Blvd., 504-522-2707

Zeitgeist Multi-Disciplinary Arts Center zeitgeistinc.net, 1618 Oretha Castle Haley Blvd., 504-827-5858

Church Alley Coffee Bar churchalleycoffeebar.tumblr.com, 1618 Oretha Castle Haley Blvd., Twitter: @churchalley

OCH Art Market ochartmarket.com, 1618 Oretha Castle Haley Blvd., 985-250-0278

Southern Food and Beverage Museum (SoFAB) sofabinstitute.org, 1504 Oretha Castle Haley Blvd., 504-569-0405

Purloo nolapurloo.com, 1504 Oretha Castle Haley Blvd., 504-324-6020

New Orleans Jazz Market 1436 Oretha Castle Haley Blvd. (still under construction as of this writing)

Southern Food and Beverage (SoFAB) Culinary Library and Archive sofabinstitute.org /sofab-culinary-library-and-archive, 1609 Oretha Castle Haley Blvd., 504-569-0405

Café Reconcile cafereconcile.org, 1631 Oretha Castle Haley Blvd., 504-568-1157

Casa Borrega casaborrega.com, 1719 Oretha Castle Haley Blvd., 504-427-0654

Charlie Boy facebook.com/charlieboynola, 2043 Oretha Castle Haley Blvd., Instagram: @charlieboynola

Roux Carré (opens 2015) goodworknetwork.org/foodcourt, 2000 Oretha Castle Haley Blvd., 504-309-2073

The Bank Architectural Antiques thebankantiques.com, 1824 Felicity St., 504-523-2702

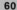

route summary

1. Begin at St. Charles Avenue and Felicity Street.
2. Facing Felicity, turn right and walk three blocks to O. C. Haley Boulevard.
3. Turn right at O. C. Haley and walk five blocks to Erato Street.
4. Cross O. C. Haley and turn left.
5. Walk seven blocks on opposite side of O. C. Haley to Josephine Street.
6. Cross O. C. Haley and turn left.
7. Walk two blocks to Felicity.
8. Turn right on Felicity and walk three blocks back to starting point on St. Charles.

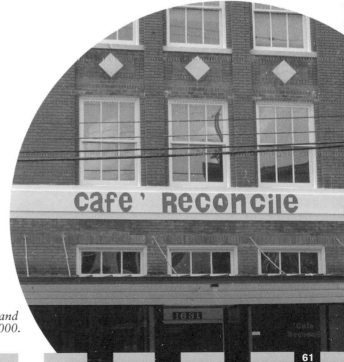

Café Reconcile has been training underserved teens and young adults in the restaurant business since 2000.

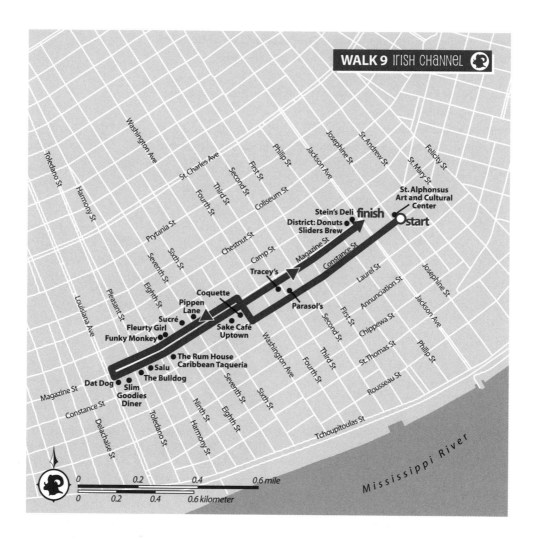

Washington Ave

Toledano St

Harmony St

St. Charles Ave

Phillip St

Jackson Ave

Josephine St

St. Andrew St

Felicity St

St. Mary St

First St

Second St

Third St

Fourth St

Prytania St

Coliseum St

Chestnut St

Camp St

St. Alphonsus Art and Cultural Center

Stein's Deli

finish

District: Donuts Sliders Brew

Magazine St

Constance St

start

Laurel St

Josephine St

Sixth St

Seventh St

Eighth St

Pleasant St

Louisiana Ave

Coquette

Pippen Lane

Sucré

Fleurty Girl

Funky Monkey

Sake Café Uptown

Tracey's

Parasol's

Annunciation St

Chippewa St

St. Thomas St

Jackson Ave

Phillip St

The Rum House Caribbean Taqueria

Salu

The Bulldog

Dat Dog

Slim Goodies Diner

Washington Ave

Seventh St

Sixth St

Fourth St

Third St

Second St

First St

Rousseau St

Magazine St

Constance St

Delachaise St

Toledano St

Ninth St

Harmony St

Eighth St

Tchoupitoulas St

Mississippi River

| 0 | 0.2 | 0.4 | 0.6 mile |

| 0 | 0.2 | 0.4 | 0.6 kilometer |

9 IRISH CHANNEL: THE LUCKIEST PLACE IN TOWN

BOUNDARIES: Constance St., Louisiana Ave., Magazine St., Jackson Ave.
DISTANCE: 2.2 miles
PARKING: Free and metered parking on the street; check signs for time limits.
PUBLIC TRANSIT: RTA Bus #11 (Magazine)

Tucked behind the elegant Garden District, the Irish Channel is a largely middle-class neighborhood whose origins date back to the early 19th century. Fearful of the potato famine that was invading their homeland, the Irish settled in the area in droves. It was an easy choice, as many boats ended up along the Mississippi River, dropping passengers off in this very area.

Although the Irish Channel is no longer predominantly Irish, the neighborhood has retained its Irish flair. It boasts some of the liveliest bars in town, including Parasol's and Tracey's. And come March, the Channel is home to the city's biggest and arguably the best St. Patrick's Day celebrations.

Among them is the Irish Channel St. Patrick's Day Club's annual Mass and parade, beginning at St. Mary's Assumption Church before green-clad revelers take to the streets on foot and by float. Parade-goers are strongly encouraged to bring along tote bags—they're likely to head home with more cabbages, potatoes, and beads than they could ever carry in their arms.

But the Irish Channel is more than just shamrocks and leprechauns. The 14-block stretch of Magazine Street between Louisiana Avenue and Jackson Avenue is a haven for shoppers and diners. And if a massage or pedicure is in your plans, there's no shortage of salons and day spas.

● **Begin your walk at 2025 Constance St., in front of the old St. Alphonsus Catholic Church, now the St. Alphonsus Art and Cultural Center. The center is maintained by the Friends of St. Alphonsus, a grassroots organization dedicated to preserving and restoring the 159-year-old church, which served the Irish Catholic community for nearly a century before it was shuttered. The center is open to the public on Tuesdays, Thursdays, and Saturdays from 10 a.m. to 2 p.m. Every March, the group presents "Fun Under the Frescoes," an Irish celebration featuring an array of musical** entertainment. St. Alphonsus Parish is now part of St. Mary's Assumption Church, just around the corner on Josephine Street.

- Walk two blocks to Jackson Avenue, cross Jackson, and continue walking on Constance, a residential area consisting of restored shotgun and camelback homes. Like so many of the neighborhoods off Magazine Street, this one has experienced a real estate boom over the past several years, its residents enjoying the ease and convenience of nearby restaurants and shops. As you walk down Constance, you may think it's Mardi Gras every day of the week, with many houses sporting decorative parade flags and fences draped with beads. Among the homes you'll pass in the first block is the one-time residence of jazz musician Dominic "Nick" LaRocca at 2218 Constance. LaRocca, a cornetist and bandleader who died in 1961, played for the group that eventually became the Original Dixieland Jazz Band.

- Walk four blocks to Third Street. The white dive of a building to the right is Parasol's, the center of the neighborhood's rollicking St. Patrick's Day festivities. The bar, which opened in 1952, is actually hopping all year long and is especially well known for its succulent roast beef po'boys.

- Walk two blocks to Washington Avenue and turn right. Walk another block to Magazine Street, cross Magazine, and turn left. Magazine stretches 6 miles, but the 14 blocks between Jackson and Louisiana Avenues boast some of the coolest, funkiest, most eclectic places in town. As you stroll along Magazine, you'll be mesmerized by the sheer variety, from Sucré, a dessert boutique between Seventh and Eighth Streets, to Funky Monkey, a secondhand-clothing and costume shop.

- Head down Magazine to Louisiana, about eight blocks. Along this stretch you'll pass Fleurty Girl, known for its New Orleans–inspired T-shirts; Bootsy's Funrock'n, dubbed a "dime store for the 21st century"; and Petcetera, a full-service pet boutique offering photography, grooming, and treats like "pupcakes" and "pet me fours."

- At Louisiana, cross Magazine, turn left, and continue walking on the opposite side of Magazine. Over the next 14 blocks, you'll likely be tempted by the many eateries that line the street. Among them are Dat Dog, a gourmet hot dog joint; Salu, a wine bar and tapas restaurant; Coquette, named in 2014 to *Southern Living*'s 100 Places to

Eat Now; The Bulldog, an international beer tavern; and The Rum House, a Caribbean taqueria. For breakfast or brunch, try Slim Goodies Diner.

● From The Rum House, at Magazine and Ninth Street, walk another 10 blocks to Jackson Avenue. Along this stretch, you'll pass Pippen Lane, an upscale children's clothing store owned by Anna Beth Goodman, wife of actor John Goodman; NOLA Couture, where you can buy New Orleans–themed neckties; and Sake Café Uptown, where sushi rolls include the Fire Roll, the Po Boy Roll, and the Jazz Roll.

During this stretch, you'll also pass through one of Magazine's few residential sections, though many homes have been converted into law offices and other commercial establishments. Amid the homes is Tracey's, the neighborhood's other Irish bar. Just a block from Parasol's, Tracey's has an equally yummy roast beef po'boy, along with 20 televisions for patrons to enjoy their favorite local sports teams. Other spots worth stopping at for a bite to eat are Stein's Deli and District: Donuts Sliders Brew, on the opposite side of Magazine just off Jackson. Any of the flags catch your eye on route? Stop in at the colorful Brad and Dellwen Flag Party, at the corner of Magazine and Jackson, and you may just find a match.

POINTS OF INTEREST

St. Alphonsus Art and Cultural Center stalphonsusneworleans.org, 2025 Constance St., 504-524-8116

Parasol's parasolsbarandrestaurant.com, 2533 Constance St., 504-302-1543

Sucré shopsucre.com, 3025 Magazine St., 504-520-8311

Bootsy's Funrock'n facebook.com/funrockn.popcity, 3109 Magazine St., 504-895-4102

Fleurty Girl fleurtygirl.net, 3117 Magazine St., 504-301-2557

Funky Monkey funkymonkeynola.com, 3127 Magazine St., 504-899-5587

Petcetera petceteranola.com, 3205 Magazine St., 504-269-8711

Dat Dog datdognola.com, 3336 Magazine St., 504-324-2226

Slim Goodies Diner slimgoodiesdiner.com, 3322 Magazine St., 504-891-3447

The Bulldog bulldog.draftfreak.com, 3236 Magazine St., 504-891-1516

Salu salurestaurant.com, 3226 Magazine St., 504-371-5809

The Rum House Caribbean Taqueria rumhousenola.com, 3128 Magazine St., 504-941-7560

Pippen Lane pippenlane.com, 2930 Magazine St., 504-269-0106

NOLA Couture nolacouture.com, 2928 Magazine St., 504-319-5959

Sake Café Uptown sakecafeuptown.us, 2830 Magazine St., 504-894-0033

Coquette coquettenola.com, 2800 Magazine St., 504-265-0421

Tracey's traceysnola.com, 2604 Magazine St., 504-897-5413

District: Donuts Sliders Brew donutsandsliders.com, 2209 Magazine St., 504-570-6945

Stein's Market & Deli steinsdeli.net, 2207 Magazine St., 504-527-0771

Brad and Dellwen Flag Party 2201 Magazine St., 504-527-5211

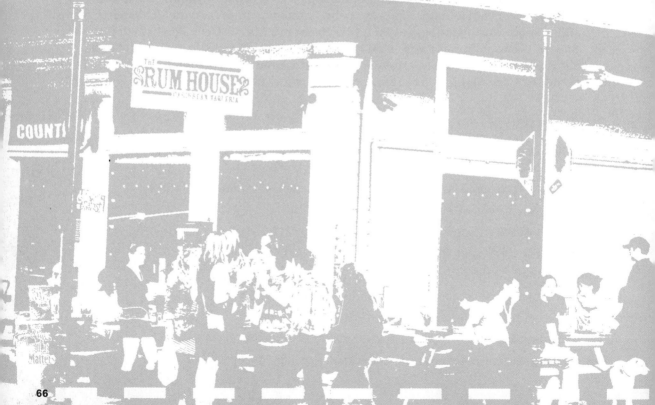

route summary

1. Begin walk at 2025 Constance St.
2. Walk two blocks to Jackson Avenue.
3. Cross Jackson and continue on Constance.
4. Walk six blocks to Washington Avenue.
5. Turn right on Washington.
6. Walk one block to Magazine.
7. Cross Magazine Street and turn left.
8. Walk eight blocks to Louisiana Avenue.
9. Cross Magazine and walk 14 blocks on opposite side of Magazine, ending at Magazine and Jackson.

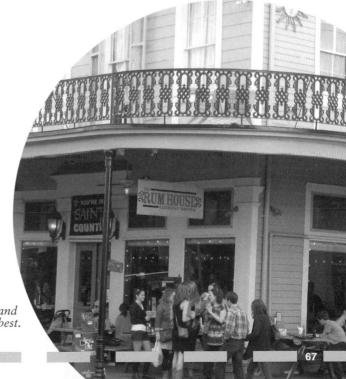

Sidewalk dining is plentiful along Magazine Street, and the island-inspired Rum House offers some of the best.

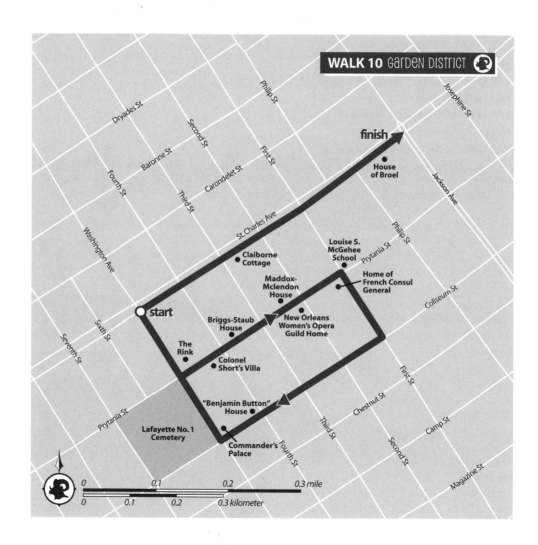

finish

House of Broel

Josephine St

Jackson Ave

Phillip St

Second St

Baronne St

Carondelet St

First St

Dryades St

Fourth St

Third St

St. Charles Ave

Washington Ave

Claiborne Cottage

Louise S. McGehee School

Prytania St

Phillip St

Coliseum St

Maddox-Mclendon House

Home of French Consul General

start

Sixth St

Briggs-Staub House

New Orleans Women's Opera Guild Home

The Rink

Colonel Short's Villa

Seventh St

First St

Prytania St

"Benjamin Button" House

Chestnut St

Camp St

Lafayette No. 1 Cemetery

Commander's Palace

Third St

Fourth St

Second St

Magazine St

0   0.1   0.2   0.3 mile

0   0.1   0.2   0.3 kilometer

10 GarDeN DISTRICT: MaNSION MaGNIFICeNCe

BOUNDARIES: St. Charles Ave., Washington Ave., Coliseum St., Jackson Ave.
DISTANCE: 1.14 miles
PARKING: Free parking on street, but some neighborhood parking is limited to 2 hours.
Check for signs.
PUBLIC TRANSIT: St. Charles Ave. Streetcar

In a city where elegance and wealth define many a neighborhood, the Garden District may well be the most enviable part of town. It includes a stretch of stately—and busy—St. Charles Avenue, but it is mostly the district's quieter and equally breathtaking interior streets that make it such an appealing place to live, or at least visit.

Listed on the National Register of Historic Places, the Garden District was developed in the early 19th century on what was once the Livaudais Plantation and several other plantations. Property was sold in parcels to wealthy Americans (specifically, WASPs) who did not want to associate with the Creoles living in the French Quarter.

The Garden District is known for its opulent Greek Revival and Italianate mansions, oak-lined streets, and, of course, magnificent gardens. It's also the neighborhood of choice for such Hollywood celebrities as John Goodman and Sandra Bullock and local luminaries such as former New Orleans Saints quarterback Archie Manning.

Most of the homes remain private residences and are therefore closed to the public. But every year, the Preservation Resource Center, a nonprofit dedicated to preserving the architecture of New Orleans, presents a self-guided holiday tour, giving the curious a chance to see up close the insides of some of the city's most beautiful homes.

● **Begin on the south side of St. Charles Avenue at Washington Avenue. Walk one block down Washington to Prytania Street. At the corner to your left is The Rink, a mini-shopping mall that includes Still Perkin', a coffeehouse; Judy at the Rink, a gift and home-decor shop; Garden District Books, one of the city's few remaining independent bookstores; and Mignon, a high-end children's clothing store. The mall gets its name from the roller-skating rink that occupied the property for the 1884 World's Fair.**

COMMANDER'S PALACE

From po'boy joints to upscale eateries, New Orleans is a city known for its restaurants. But nothing says "fine dining" quite like Commander's Palace, the Garden District establishment that Emile Commander opened in 1880 to give the neighborhood's well-heeled newcomers an incomparable dining experience.

While many restaurants have come and gone in New Orleans, Commander's, now owned by a branch of the noted Brennan family, continues to draw locals and tourists alike with its award-winning menu of modern Louisiana and Creole fare, from classic turtle soup and crispy pork belly and oysters to griddle-seared Gulf fish and bread-pudding soufflé.

In 2013, chef Tory McPhail was named Best Chef: South in the James Beard Foundation Awards, and Commander's came in fourth in TripAdvisor's list of Travelers' Favorite Fine-Dining Restaurants–United States. *Business Insider* named it one of the 45 Best Restaurants in America, and it made *Southern Living* magazine's list of 100 Places to Eat Now.

Commander's is pricey, so if money is an object, here's a tip: Go for lunch and take advantage of the two-course lunch specials ($17–$22) and 25¢ martinis. If you're celebrating a special occasion, the weekend jazz brunch is as festive as it gets. Before you go, be sure to check **commanders palace.com** for the dress code.

● Cross Prytania Street at Washington, turn left, and walk one block to Fourth Street. At the corner, 1448 Fourth, is Colonel Short's Villa, built in 1859 for Col. Robert Henry Short, a cotton merchant. The cast-iron fence surrounding the home features patterns of cornstalks and morning glories; legend has it that Short bought the fence for his wife because she missed her home state of Iowa. The Italianate-style mansion was built by architect Henry Howard, who designed some of Louisiana's most elegant homes, including Nottaway, Louisiana's largest plantation.

● Cross Fourth Street and continue walking down Prytania. At 2605 Prytania, at the corner of Third and Prytania, is the Briggs-Staub House, which was built in 1849 and is the only example of Gothic Revival architecture in the Garden District.

- Cross Third Street. Across the street, at 2523 Prytania, is the old Our Mother of Perpetual Help, a one-time chapel that best-selling author Anne Rice attended as a child and later bought and converted to a private residence. At more than 13,000 square feet, the house was said to be too small for Rice, who went on to buy and renovate an old orphanage on nearby Napoleon Avenue. Actor Nicolas Cage once owned not only this house but also the LaLaurie House in the Lower French Quarter (see Walk 5), but he lost both to foreclosure in 2009.

- Continue walking to 2507 Prytania, the Maddox-Mclendon House, a Greek Revival mansion built for Joseph H. Maddox, owner of the *New Orleans Daily Crescent* newspaper, in the 1850s. The interior, which was used in the Jamie Foxx–Leonardo DiCaprio movie *Django Unchained,* features a grand staircase made of mahogany, cypress, and walnut; Baccarat crystal chandeliers; and an opulent ballroom with hand-painted ceilings, among other amenities.

  At 2504 Prytania is the New Orleans Women's Opera Guild Home, which was built in 1859 for Edward A. Davis and donated to the Women's Guild of the New Orleans Opera Association in 1965. The Greek Revival home was designed by noted architect William A. Freret and is open for public tours on Mondays.

- Walk one block to 2406 Prytania, the home of French consul general Grégor Trumel and his family. Built in 1905 by attorney John May, the Colonial Revival house was purchased by the Republic of France in 1957 and has housed its consul ever since. According to the Preservation Resource Center, it has undergone numerous renovations over the years but continues to operate as a symbol of the connection and commitment between Louisiana and France.

- Cross First Street. The house directly across Prytania is the Bradish Johnson House, a one-time private residence that now serves as the main building for Louise S. McGehee School, an independent girls' school. The house was designed by James Freret and built in 1872 for wealthy sugar magnate Bradish Johnson. Today, it houses McGehee libraries, classrooms, and the office of the headmistress.

- Turn right on First Street. In the middle of the block, at 1420 First St., is the home of former New Orleans Saints quarterback Archie Manning. It is also the childhood home of Manning's three sons, including NFL quarterbacks Peyton and Eli Manning. An ESPN documentary, *The Book of Manning,* tells the story of growing up Manning and features scenes of father and sons tossing the football in the front yard.

- Walk one block to Coliseum Street and turn right. At 2425 Coliseum is the Joseph Merrick Jones House, home of actor John Goodman and the former home of Nine Inch Nails singer Trent Reznor. The house is named for a lawyer who lived there in the mid-1900s. Joseph Merrick Jones also served as secretary for public affairs for the US State Department during World War II and as president of Tulane University.

- Walk two block to 2627 Coliseum, a Swiss chalet–style mansion built in 1876 by architect William Freret for James Eustis, a US senator and ambassador to France. Today, the house is owned by Academy Award–winning actress Sandra Bullock, whose ties to New Orleans go back to Hurricane Katrina in 2005. Following the storm, Bullock adopted the heavily damaged Warren Easton Charter High School in Mid-City and has played a significant role in the school's subsequent success. While in New Orleans, she adopted her son, Louis, and in 2010 bought the Coliseum Street mansion.

- In the next block, at 2707 Coliseum, stands the so-called Benjamin Button House, the primary residence used in the Brad Pitt–Cate Blanchett film *The Curious Case of Benjamin Button.* The Academy Award–winning movie, based on the short story by F. Scott Fitzgerald, was filmed almost entirely in New Orleans. The 8,000-square-foot white center-hall cottage was built in 1832 and has been owned by three generations of the Nolan family. In the movie it served as the old folks' home where Queenie, the resident manager played by Taraji P. Henson, raises Button, who, of course, was played by Pitt.

- Continue walking down Coliseum to the corner of Washington Avenue. The mammoth turquoise structure on the right is the legendary Commander's Palace, a fine-dining institution renowned not just in New Orleans but worldwide. Owned today by noted restaurateur Ella Brennan, it dates back to 1880, when Emile Commander opened the only restaurant patronized by the Garden District's distinguished families. Known for its modern Louisiana and Creole cuisine—with Sunday jazz brunch among its most popular meals—Commander's has won countless accolades (see sidebar).

- Cross Washington Avenue and turn right. You're now in front of Lafayette No. 1 Cemetery, established in 1833 in what used to be known as the city of Lafayette.

The cemetery is dedicated to musician Theodore Von LaHache, who founded the New Orleans Philharmonic Society. Among those buried here are Confederate general Harry T. Hayes and Civil War–era Louisiana governor Henry Watkins Allen. Scenes from the movie *Interview with the Vampire* were filmed here. The entrance is a half-block down on Washington Avenue. Feel free to stroll through the cemetery— lots of people do—and then return to the entrance.

● Walk one block to St. Charles Avenue and turn right. Continue walking to 2618 St. Charles. Known as the Belfort Mansion, this 19th-century Greek Revival home housed seven strangers in the 2000 edition of the MTV reality show *The Real World: New Orleans.* (The series filmed again in New Orleans in 2010, this time housing its cast on Dufossat Street in Uptown.)

● Walk another block to 2524 St. Charles to the Greek Revival home known as the Claiborne Cottage. Anne Rice lived here as a teenager, and the home is the setting for her book *Violin.*

● Continue walking to 2220 St. Charles. The House of Broel was built in the 1850s by George Washington Squires. The house, which today is used as a wedding and party venue, features the Mystic Ballroom, a lavish setting with ornate chandeliers and original black-marble fireplaces. The house is open for public tours.

● Walk to the corner of St. Charles and Jackson Avenue. Your tour ends here.

POINTS OF INTEREST

Garden District Book Shop gardendistrictbookshop.com, 2727 Prytania St., 504-895-2266

Still Perkin' neworleanscoffeeshop.com, 2727 Prytania St., 504-899-0335

Judy at the Rink facebook.com/judyattherink, 2727 Prytania St., 504-891-7018

Mignon mignonnola.com, 2727 Prytania St., 504-891-2374

New Orleans Women's Opera Guild Home operaguildhome.org, 2504 Prytania St., 504-899-1945

Louise S. McGehee School mcgeheeschool.com, 2343 Prytania St., 504-561-1224

Commander's Palace commanderspalace.com, 1403 Washington Ave., 504-899-8221

Lafayette No. 1 Cemetery saveourcemeteries.org/lafayette-cemetery-no-1,
1400 Washington Ave., 504-658-3781

House of Broel houseofbroel.com, 2220 St. Charles Ave., 504-522-2220

route summary

1. Begin walk at St. Charles Avenue and Washington Avenue.
2. Walk one block to Prytania St.
3. Cross Prytania and turn left.
4. Walk four blocks to First Street and turn right.
5. Walk one block to Coliseum Street and turn right.
6. Walk four blocks to Washington Avenue and turn right.
7. Walk one block to St. Charles Avenue and turn right.
8. Walk six blocks to Jackson Avenue.

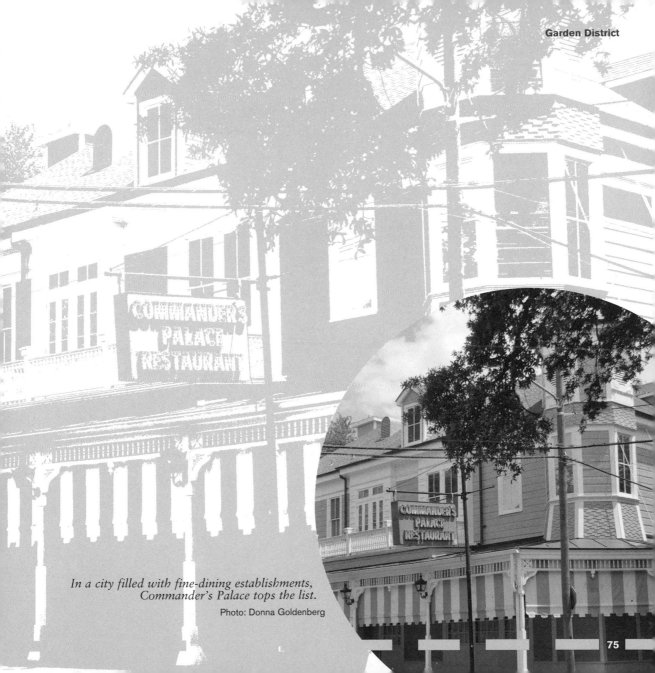

*In a city filled with fine-dining establishments,
Commander's Palace tops the list.*

Photo: Donna Goldenberg

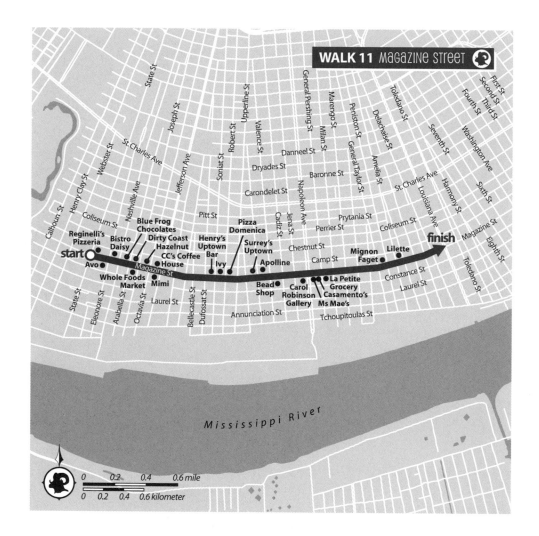

start

finish

Reginelli's
Pizzeria

Avo

Bistro
Daisy

Blue Frog
Chocolates

Dirty Coast

Hazelnut

CC's Coffee
House

Whole Foods
Market

Mimi

Henry's
Uptown
Bar

Ivy

Pizza
Domenica

Surrey's
Uptown

Apolline

Bead
Shop

Carol
Robinson
Gallery

La Petite
Grocery

Casamento's

Ms Mae's

Mignon
Faget

Lilette

Magazine St

State St

Henry Clay St

Webster St

Coliseum St

Calhoun St

St. Charles Ave

Nashville Ave

Joseph St

Jefferson Ave

State St

Eleonore St

Arabella St

Octavia St

Laurel St

Bellecastle St

Dufossat St

Pitt St

Soniat St

Robert St

Valence St

Upperline St

Annunciation St

Danneel St

Dryades St

Carondelet St

Baronne St

General Pershing St

Marengo St

Milan St

Peniston St

Delachaise St

General Taylor St

Napoleon Ave

Cadiz St

Jena St

Prytania St

Perrier St

Chestnut St

Camp St

Constance St

Laurel St

Tchoupitoulas St

Amelia St

St. Charles Ave

Coliseum St

Louisiana Ave

Toledano St

Seventh St

Harmony St

Washington Ave

Fourth St

Third St

Second St

First St

Sixth St

Magazine St

Eighth St

Toledano St

Mississippi River

0   0.2   0.4   0.6 mile

0   0.2   0.4   0.6 kilometer

11 Magazine Street: From Chic to Cheap

BOUNDARIES: **Magazine St., Louisiana Ave., State St.**
DISTANCE: **2 miles**
PARKING: **Metered parking on Magazine; free in the neighborhood, but check signs for time limits.**
PUBLIC TRANSIT: **RTA Bus #11 (Magazine). For $3 you can buy a Jazzy Pass, which lets you take unlimited bus rides in a single day.**

In a city brimming with cool streets, from funky Frenchmen Street in Faubourg Marigny to ritzy Royal Street in the French Quarter, none may be cooler than Magazine Street, a 6-mile stretch that runs from Audubon Park to the Central Business District.

Magazine has it all, from high-end boutiques to secondhand stores, from po'boy joints to fine-dining bistros, and from sports bars to music clubs. There are yoga studios, art galleries, and antiques stores, not to mention day spas, coffeehouses, and dessert cafés.

Two Mardi Gras parades—Muses and Thoth—roll on portions of Magazine, as does the Irish Channel St. Patrick's Day Parade. Other events on Magazine include Art for Arts' Sake, a gallery-hopping affair signaling the start of the fall arts season. The annual Champagne Stroll, held the Saturday evening before Mother's Day, gives last-minute shoppers a chance to buy the perfect gift for Mom.

Magazine follows the length of the Mississippi River crescent and takes in such neighborhoods as Uptown, the Garden District, the Irish Channel, the Warehouse District, and Downtown. Because Magazine is also included in our Lower Garden District and Irish Channel tours (Walks 7 and 9, respectively), this walk is limited to the stretch between State Street and Louisiana Avenue in Uptown.

● **Begin at the corner of State and Magazine, in front of Reginelli's, a popular New Orleans pizza chain, and across the street from Noodle & Pie, one of the city's newest eateries. In the first couple of blocks, you'll pass several other restaurants, including the upscale-yet-casual Avo and Bistro Daisy, housed in a quaint yellow** cottage. Avo, which opens in the spring of 2015, will specialize in Italian cuisine; Bistro Daisy serves French food with a Southern twist.

- Cross Nashville Avenue and continue down Magazine. Got a sweet tooth? Stop at Blue Frog Chocolates (5707 Magazine), known for its confections from around the world. If you're in the market for a New Orleans T-shirt, check out Dirty Coast (5631 Magazine). You won't find X-rated T-shirts here—for those, you'll have to head to Bourbon Street. What you will find are some of the cleverest, most New Orleans–centric shirts in town. Examples include "One Nation Under Dome" (in reference to Saints and the Superdome), "504ever" (in reference to the city's area code), and "Death by Crawfish."

The mammoth building to your right is Whole Foods Market, which when it was being developed in 2001 met with a mix of reactions, from euphoria to rage. Opponents argued the store would be too big for the neighborhood; supporters liked the idea of developing a blighted but historic building, the old Arabella bus barn. Today, it's hard to imagine this block without Whole Foods, where if you're lucky you might just see New Orleans Saints quarterback Drew Brees—who lives in the 'hood—pushing a cart. And with so many movies being filmed in New Orleans these days, celebrity sightings aren't uncommon: Will Ferrell, Emma Roberts, and Sarah Jessica Parker have shopped here, and Whole Foods was also one of the stomping grounds of the *Top Chef: New Orleans* cast.

- The next two blocks, between Joseph Street and Jefferson Avenue, are chock-full of unique and fun shops. Among them are Hazelnut, a home-decor store co-owned by local celebrity and former *Mad Men* actor Bryan Batt; Plum, which sells "cool stuff for stylish living"; and EarthSavers, known for its luxurious spa treatments. Azby's, Mimi, Jean Therapy, and Spring are just a few of the area's upscale boutiques. If you're bargain-hunting, head to Swap, a consignment store billed as a "haven for fashion-able and budget-conscious women." Haus 131 also has reasonably priced apparel.

- Cross Jefferson at CC's Coffee House. To your right is Poydras Home, a nursing home and assisted-living center founded in 1817 as a home for women and children left widowed and orphaned by the yellow fever epidemic. Named for business-man and philanthropist Julien Poydras (see Walk 3), it moved to its present site on

Magazine in 1857. The next stretch of blocks is largely residential, though you will pass a handful of businesses, such as Guy's Po-Boys, where you can get a roast beef topped with fries and Cheddar cheese (we kid you not), and Tee-Eva's Old Fashioned Pies and Pralines, which has been featured in numerous magazines as well as on the Travel Channel and the Food Network.

- At 5116 Magazine, between Soniat and Dufossat Streets, is St. Katharine Drexel Preparatory School, a Catholic girls' school that until the 2013–14 academic year had been the century-old Xavier Preparatory School, run by the Sisters of the Blessed Sacrament. Because of financial issues, the sisters announced they were closing after 98 years of educating primarily African American girls. Determined to keep the school open, a group of Xavier Prep alumni purchased the campus and led the way for its transformation to St. Katharine Drexel Prep.

- At the corner of Sonlat and Magazine is Henry's Uptown Bar, a century-old institution that, according to legend, was a favorite watering hole of JFK assassin Lee Harvey Oswald, who was born and raised in New Orleans. In its coverage of the 50th anniversary of JFK's assassination, *The Times-Picayune* wrote extensively about Oswald's time in New Orleans, including the story of him being thrown out of Henry's when the owner refused to turn on the television coverage of his arrest for passing out "Hands Off Cuba" pamphlets on Canal Street.

- In the next block is Ivy, one of the city's newest upscale eateries. The chef is Sue Zemanick, who also runs the kitchen at nearby Gautreau's, another of the city's top-rated restaurants. In 2014, Zemanick tied with Ryan Prewitt, chef of Pêche Seafood Grill in the Warehouse District (see Walk 1), for Best Chef: South in the prestigious James Beard Foundation Awards. A block from Ivy is Pizza Domenica, the casual offshoot of chef John Besh's Domenica in the Roosevelt Hotel downtown (see Walk 2, Canal Street).

- For breakfast or lunch, check out Surrey's Uptown. The place is generally packed, but the wait for such dishes as huevos rancheros, crabmeat omelets, or fried green tomatoes is worth it. Just next door, at the corner of Bordeaux Street and Magazine, is Le Bon Temps Roulé, another classic Uptown bar. *Laissez les bons temps rouler* means "Let the good times roll," and this live-music venue lives up to its name, serving free oysters on Fridays and $1 beers during Saints games. The Soul Rebels, a New Orleans brass band, performs on Thursday nights.

Other restaurants scattered over the next several blocks include Fare Food Apothecary, a health-food café; McClure's Barbecue, named one of New Orleans's 10 hottest restaurants by Zagat; and Apolline, an upscale Southern bistro where you can have a drink custom-made to suit your mood and taste. For $25, you get a consultation and two drinks, and your special recipe is stored for future visits.

Several boutiques can be found on this stretch as well, from Jezebel's, which sells vintage costume jewelry and antique fabrics, to the Bead Shop, which carries an amazing inventory of beads and beading supplies and has a stringing room where you can make your own necklace, bracelet, or earrings. If you're a beginner, one of the store's beading experts will walk you through the process.

● Walk to the corner of Magazine and Napoleon. To the right, facing Napoleon, is the Carol Robinson Gallery, which operates out of a restored 19th-century house. It features the works of such artists as Mississippi painters Jere Allen and Robert Malone, sculptor Ron Dale, Japanese painter Masahiro Arai, local pastel artists Sandra Burshell and Ed Dyer, and abstract painters Bernard Mattox and Karen Jacobs. Also on display are three-dimensional works, including Roddy Capers's blown-glass vases and Michael Yankowski's wooden altarpieces.

● Cross Napoleon Avenue and continue walking down Magazine. To your right is Ms. Mae's, a 24-hour dive known for cheap drinks. During the 2013 NFL football season, it was also a favorite hangout of Saints defensive coordinator Rob Ryan, who twice bought rounds of drinks for fans in celebration of victories over the hated Atlanta Falcons and the Dallas Cowboys, the team that had fired him a year earlier.

● To the left is Lawrence Square, where at almost any time of the day you'll see a rousing game of basketball; and the Second District headquarters of the New Orleans Police Department. Next to the police station is St. George's, an independent Episcopal school founded in 1969.

● Across Magazine and next to Ms. Mae's is the legendary oyster house Casamento's, established in 1919 by Italian immigrant Joe Casamento. The place is known as much for its tile decor as it is for its fried-oyster loaves. If you're in the market for a tutu or tiara, stop in at the Uptown Costume Shop, which also stocks a bounty of masks, wigs, and feather boas, not to mention Elvis apparel.

● Walk one block to the corner of Magazine and General Pershing Street. To the right is the highly rated La Petite Grocery, whose owner and executive chef, Justin Devillier, was a contestant on Bravo TV's *Top Chef: New Orleans.* The building once housed a full-service grocery store with a barn in the back to house delivery carriages. Devillier, who's won much acclaim for his culinary creativity (can you say blue-crab beignets?), was named a James Beard Award finalist in 2012, 2013, and 2014 for Best Chef: South.

● Walk two blocks to the corner of Marengo Street, where you'll see Neal Auction Company to the right. Established in 1983, it holds auctions six times a year, with each comprising fine art and antiques from estates, private collections, and cultural institutions. During the next stretch, you'll pass several high-end clothing boutiques, including the Uptown shop of New Orleans jewelry designer Mignon Faget, at the corner of Magazine and Peniston.

● Yet another award-winning restaurant, the French- and Italian-inspired Lilette, has sat at the corner of Magazine and Antonine since 2000. Housed in a one-time apothecary, Lilette was once dubbed "the sexiest dining room in New Orleans" by *Travel & Leisure* magazine. Owner and chef John Harris has been named a James Beard finalist for Best Chef: South, and in 2002, *Food & Wine* named him one of the best new chefs in America.

● In the next block, at 3606 Magazine St., is the home of WRBH, the city's radio station for the blind and visually impaired. The station's mission is "to turn the written word into the spoken word so that the blind and print handicapped receive the same ease of access to current information as their sighted peers." WRBH is the only full-time reading service on the FM dial in the United States, and one of only three in the world. Because of the station's streaming capability, it reaches people worldwide.

● Walk three blocks to Louisiana Avenue and catch RTA Bus #11 for your trip back to the starting point. Of course, if you're up to it, feel free to walk beyond Louisiana before making the trek back.

POINTS OF INTEREST

Reginelli's Pizzeria reginellis.com, 5961 Magazine St., 504-899-1414

Avo (opens spring 2015) 5908 Magazine St.

Bistro Daisy bistrodaisy.com, 5831 Magazine St., 504-899-6987

Blue Frog Chocolates bluefrogchocolates.com, 5707 Magazine St., 504-269-5707

Dirty Coast dirtycoast.com, 5631 Magazine St., 504-324-3745

Hazelnut hazelnutneworleans.com, 5515 Magazine St., 504-891-2424

Whole Foods Market–Arabella Station wholefoodsmarket.com/stores/arabellastation, 5600 Magazine St., 504-899-9119

EarthSavers earthsaversonline.com, 5501 Magazine St., 504-899-8555

Spring springboutique.net, 5525 Magazine St., 504-896-9185

Mimi miminola.com, 5500 Magazine St., 504-269-6464

CC's Coffee House ccscoffeehouse.com, 900 Jefferson Ave., 504-891-4969

Henry's Uptown Bar facebook.com/henrys.uptown.bar, 5101 Magazine St., 504-324-8140

Ivy ivynola.com, 5015 Magazine St., 504-899-1330

Pizza Domenica pizzadomenica.com, 4933 Magazine St., 504-301-4978

Surrey's Uptown surreycafeandjuicebar.com, 4807 Magazine St., 504-895-5757

Le Bon Temps Roulé 4801 Magazine St., 504-895-8117

Apolline apollinerestaurant.com, 4729 Magazine St., 504-894-8869

Bead Shop beadshopneworleans.com, 4612 Magazine St., 504-895-6161

Carol Robinson Gallery carolrobinsongallery.com, 840 Napoleon Ave., 504-895-6130

Ms. Mae's msmaeswallofshame.blogspot.com, 4336 Magazine St., 504-218-8035

Casamento's casamentosrestaurant.com, 4330 Magazine St., 504-895-9761

La Petite Grocery lapetitegrocery.com, 4238 Magazine St., 504-891-3377

Mignon Faget mignonfaget.com, 3801 Magazine St., 504-891-2005

Lilette liletterestaurant.com, 3637 Magazine St., 504-895-1636

route summary

1. Begin walk at Magazine Street and State Street.
2. Walk 32 blocks to Louisiana Avenue.

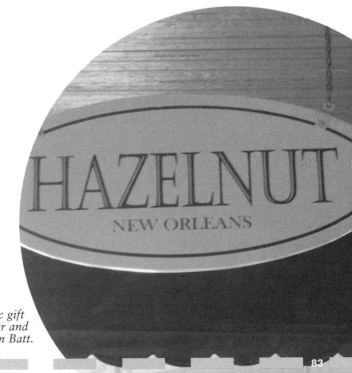

Need a wedding gift? Head to Hazelnut, a chic gift shop co-owned by former Mad Men *star and New Orleans native Bryan Batt.*

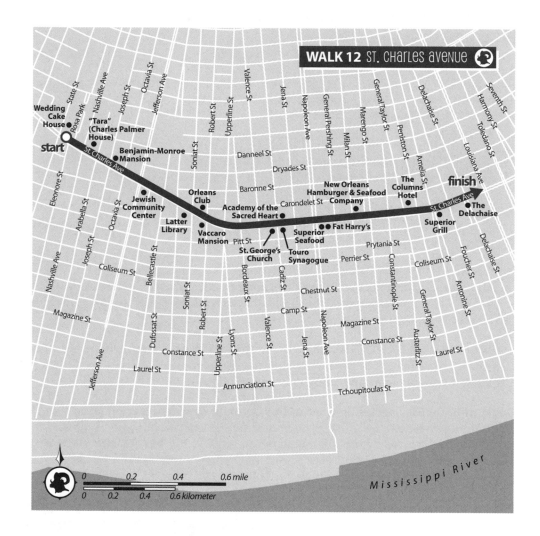

WALK 12 ST. Charles avenue

Wedding Cake House

"Tara" (Charles Palmer House)

start

Benjamin-Monroe Mansion

Jewish Community Center

Orleans Club

Latter Library

Vaccaro Mansion

Academy of the Sacred Heart

St. George's Church

Superior Seafood

Touro Synagogue

Fat Harry's

New Orleans Hamburger & Seafood Company

The Columns Hotel

finish

Superior Grill

The Delachaise

State St
Rosa Park
Nashville Ave
Joseph St
Octavia St
Jefferson Ave
St. Charles Ave
Eleonore St
Arabella St
Octavia St
Soniat St
Robert St
Upperline St
Valence St
Jena St
Napoleon Ave
General Pershing St
General Taylor St
Marengo St
Milan St
Penistron St
Delachaise St
Amelia St
Seventh St
Harmony St
Toledano St
Louisiana Ave
St. Charles Ave

Danneel St
Dryades St
Baronne St
Carondelet St
Prytania St
Perrier St
Constantinople St
Coliseum St
Foucher St
Delachaise St
Antonine St

Nashville Ave
Joseph St
Coliseum St
Bellecastle St
Soniat St
Robert St
Pitt St
Cadiz St
Chestnut St
Camp St
General Taylor St
Austerlitz St
Laurel St

Magazine St
Dufossat St
Constance St
Laurel St
Upperline St
Lyons St
Valence St
Jena St
Napoleon Ave
Magazine St
Constance St

Jefferson Ave
Annunciation St
Tchoupitoulas St

Mississippi River

0   0.2   0.4   0.6 mile
0   0.2   0.4   0.6 kilometer

84

12 ST. CHARLES AVENUE: JEWEL OF NEW ORLEANS

BOUNDARIES: St. Charles Ave., Louisiana Ave., Eleonore St.
DISTANCE: 2.77 miles
PARKING: Free on St. Charles and in the surrounding neighborhood, but bear in mind that parking on some residential streets is limited to 2 hours.
PUBLIC TRANSIT: St. Charles Avenue Streetcar

If there's one street in New Orleans that's made for walking, it's magnificent St. Charles Avenue, the so-called Jewel of America's Grand Avenues and one of the top 10 thoroughfares in the United States as ranked by the American Planning Association in 2007.

Stretching 6.4 miles from the Central Business District to Riverbend, St. Charles Avenue is known for its exquisite mansions, many of which date back to the mid-19th century, when it became home to New Orleans's wealthiest and most powerful citizens.

Most of the mansions still stand today, though some have been converted to luxury apartment buildings, bed-and-breakfasts, or in one case a public library. Numerous churches, synagogues, schools, and businesses, along with Tulane and Loyola Universities and Audubon Park, also make their homes on the grand, oak-lined avenue.

The best way to see St. Charles Avenue is on foot or by streetcar, so the following walking tour allows for both. Take your time as you marvel at the avenue's beauty, then hop on the streetcar, grab a window seat, and enjoy the view once again.

● **Begin at 5809 St. Charles, in front of the Colonial Revival mansion known as the Wedding Cake House because of its many layers and adornments. Probably the most photographed house on the avenue, it dates back to the late 19th century, when it served as the home of Nicholas Burke, a wholesale grocer. The house has undergone numerous renovations and was rebuilt in 1907 after an electrical fire.**

● **Walk one block, cross Nashville Avenue, and check out the George Palmer House at 5705 St. Charles. Though not nearly as large as most of the mansions on the avenue, the plantation-style house is famous for being built to resemble Tara, the O'Hara**

Latter Library

With its lavish grounds and neo-Italianate design, the mansion between Dufossat and Soniat streets fits in perfectly with the other palatial homes along St. Charles Ave. But instead of housing people, it houses books.

Listed on the National Register of Historic Places, the Milton H. Latter Memorial Library was built in the early 20th century as the private residence of Mark Isaacs, founder of Maison Blanche, one of the city's legendary department stores.

When Isaacs died in 1912, lumber magnate Frank B. Williams bought the house. His son Harry Williams, an aviation pioneer, was married to Marguerite Clark, an American stage and silent-film actress. The couple inherited the house after the elder Williams's death and lived there until 1936, when Harry Williams died in a plane crash. Clark lived there for another three years before moving to New York.

Racetrack owner Robert Eddy bought the house in 1937, and a decade later, he sold it to real estate executive Harry Latter. Looking for a way to memorialize their only son, Milton, who was killed in World War II, Latter and his wife immediately donated it to the city for use as a public library.

Although the library has undergone numerous renovations over the years, it has preserved many of the formal rooms as reading rooms, along with some of the home's original adornments, among them Czechoslovakian chandeliers, Dutch murals, and South American mahogany paneling.

Regular events at Latter include book sales, film screenings, author visits, summer reading programs, early-literacy events, and adult programming. The library is open seven days a week, so be sure to stop in for a visit while walking the avenue. Call 504-596-2625 or visit **tinyurl .com/nolapubliclibraries** for hours.

family home in *Gone with the Wind.* Another historic house once stood at this site; it was built for Lawrence Fabacher, who founded Jax Brewery (see Walk 6).

● Walk two blocks to the Benjamin-Monroe Mansion at 5531 St. Charles. The 22-room Italianate Beaux Arts Renaissance Revival house was designed by noted New Orleans architect Emile Weil for businessman Emmanuel V. Benjamin in 1912. It was later owned by J. Edgar Monroe, a shipbuilder and philanthropist, followed by several other owners. Next to the Benjamin-Monroe house is Danneel Playspot, one of the city's nearly 120 parks and playgrounds.

● Walk one block and cross Jefferson Avenue. To the right, at 5342 St. Charles, is the Jewish Community Center, which has occupied the corner of St. Charles and Jefferson since 1948. The JCC actually dates back to 1855 with the formation of the Young Men's Hebrew and Literary Society. The society eventually became the Young Men's Hebrew Association and later the Young Men's and Young Women's Hebrew Association. It changed its name to the Jewish Community Center upon moving to its current location, the site of the former Jewish Children's Home. The JCC offers an array of programming, from summer camp and nursery school to health-and-wellness activities and Jewish holiday celebrations.

Next to the JCC, at 5300 St. Charles, is De La Salle High School, home of the Cavaliers, which was founded as a Catholic School for boys in 1949 but which became coed in 1992. De La Salle is part of the Brothers of the Christian Schools network, which has 1,500 schools in 85 countries.

● Walk one block to Dufossat Street. To the right, at 5120 St. Charles, is the Milton H. Latter Memorial Library, a former private home that is undoubtedly the most stunning of the New Orleans Public Library's 14 branches (see sidebar).

● Walk one block to 5010 St. Charles. The Tudor-style house was built in 1909 for Joseph Vaccaro, founder of the Standard Fruit and Steamship Company, one of the first businesses to import bananas from Honduras to New Orleans. Standard Fruit eventually became the Dole Food Company.

To the left, at 5005 St. Charles, is the home of the Orleans Club, an exclusive women's club. Built in 1868 as a wedding gift from Colonel William Lewis Wynn to his only daughter, Ann Elizabeth Wynn Garner. The house remained in private hands until 1925, when a group of 300 women purchased it for a club dedicated to women's interests and the arts. Today, members host a variety of cultural-arts programs along with debutante teas and other society functions.

- Walk three blocks to 4717 St. Charles. The Richardsonian Romanesque Revival mansion is easily one of the largest houses on the Avenue, at 22,000 square feet and four stories. It was built over three years in the early 20th century by cotton magnate W. P. Brown, founder of Hibernia Bank, as a wedding gift for his wife. In 2011, two floors of the house were open to the public for the first time as part of a tour to benefit the New Orleans Museum of Art.

- Walk one block to St. George's Episcopal Church (4600 St. Charles), which got its start as a diocesan mission just before the Civil War at the corner of Berlin (now General Pershing Street) and Magazine Streets. The present-day church was dedicated in 1900, its architecture and stained-glass windows among its most noted features. In 1969, church leaders opened St. George's Episcopal School on nearby Camp Street. One of the school buildings is located on the site of the original mission. Among other programs, the church hosts the Dragon Café, which serves free breakfast every Sunday morning to the hungry and poor.

- Walk another block to 4534 St. Charles. The stone Mediterranean-style villa was built in 1906 for William Mason Smith, president of the New Orleans Cotton Exchange. To the left, at 4521 St. Charles, is the Academy of the Sacred Heart, a Catholic girls' school that is part of a network of Sacred Heart schools around the world. Sacred Heart dates back to the early 19th century, when it was based in the French Quarter. In 1847 it moved to a Greek Revival mansion on St. Charles, to accommodate the growing number of families who were moving Uptown. When that building proved to be too small, a new Colonial Revival–style structure went up in its place in 1900. Over the years, the school has undergone numerous renovations and expansions—so many, in fact, that the only remnant of its origins is a wrought-iron fountain topped with a swan.

- Continue walking down St. Charles and cross at Napoleon Avenue. To the left are the Sacred Heart nursery school, preschool, and primary school, known as the Mater Campus, which opened in 2005. To the right are Superior Seafood and Fat Harry's, a legendary watering hole. During Carnival season, this intersection is one of the most popular places for parade-watching, with dozens of parades making the turn onto St. Charles from Napoleon. One thing you're sure to notice as you continue down St. Charles are all the beads hanging from the trees, the result of float riders missing their targets on the streets. On Fat Tuesday, as well as the days leading up to it, the streets are wall-to-wall people, especially for such parades as Bacchus, Orpheus, Muses, and Rex.

- Walk another block to 4238 St. Charles, home of Touro Synagogue, the sixth oldest synagogue in the country and the first outside the 13 original colonies. On the first Friday of the New Orleans Jazz & Heritage Festival, Touro, a Reform synagogue, sponsors Jazz Fest Shabbat, a rousing Sabbath service featuring some of the city's top musicians along with the temple's choir and cantor.

- In the next block, at 4141 St. Charles, is New Orleans Hamburger & Seafood Company, part of a local chain of casual eateries where you can also get beignets. Back in the 1980s, the building housed 4141, one of the city's most popular discos.

- Walk three blocks to The Columns (3811 St. Charles), a boutique hotel in a late-19th-century Italianate house designed by Thomas Sully, considered one of New Orleans's greatest architects. Listed in the National Register of Historic Places, The Columns was once the home of cigar magnate Simon Hernsheim. Featuring a grand mahogany staircase and many other original details, it later became a boardinghouse, and, in 1953, a hotel. If time allows, stop in for a drink in the Victorian Lounge, once the main dining room, or enjoy a bite to eat on the grand veranda. Several movies and TV shows have been shot here, including Brooke Shields's 1978 film debut, *Pretty Baby*, and the popular FX anthology series *American Horror Story: Coven*.

- As you continue walking down St. Charles, you'll pass numerous luxury condo developments. At 3636 St. Charles is Superior Grill, a Mexican restaurant known for its happy hours and for being a popular gathering spot for Mardi Gras parades. The best seats in the house are on the patio, where you can watch the streetcars roll by over a plate of crawfish enchiladas and a frozen margarita. Equally fun but with a different vibe is The Delachaise, a wine bar at 3442 St. Charles. The outdoor patio, with its twinkling lights, is the perfect spot to share a bottle of wine and a cheese plate.

- The walk officially ends at St. Charles and Louisiana Avenue, but feel free to continue the stroll—until your feet give out—and catch the streetcar back to the starting point. The St. Charles Ave. Streetcar was recently named a National Historic Landmark and is well worth the experience.

POINTS OF INTEREST

Danneel Playspot 5501 St. Charles Ave. at Octavia Street

Jewish Community Center nojcc.org, 5342 St. Charles Ave., 504-897-0143

Milton H. Latter Memorial Library tinyurl.com/nolapubliclibraries, 5120 St. Charles Ave., 504-596-2625

Academy of the Sacred Heart ashrosary.org, 4521 St. Charles Ave., 504-891-1943

Superior Seafood superiorseafoodnola.com, 4338 St. Charles Ave., 504-293-3474

Touro Synagogue tourosynagogue.com, 4238 St. Charles Ave., 504-895-4843

New Orleans Hamburger & Seafood Company nohsc.com, 4141 St. Charles Ave., 504-247-9753

Fat Harry's fatharrysneworleans.com, 4330 St. Charles Ave., 504-895-9582

The Columns Hotel thecolumns.com, 3811 St. Charles Ave., 504-899-9308

Superior Grill superiorgrill.com, 3636 St. Charles Ave., 504-899-4200

The Delachaise thedelachaise.com, 3442 St. Charles Ave., 504-895-0858

route summary

1. Begin walk at 5809 St. Charles Avenue, between State Street and Rosa Park.
2. Walk 27 blocks to Louisiana Avenue.

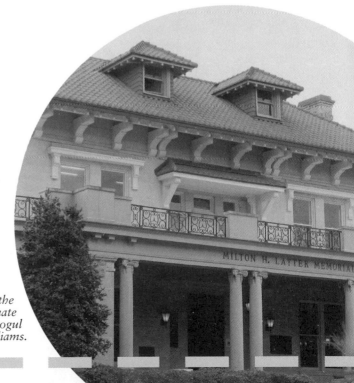

The Milton H. Latter Memorial Library was the onetime residence of department store magnate Mark Isaacs and later lumber mogul Frank B. Williams.

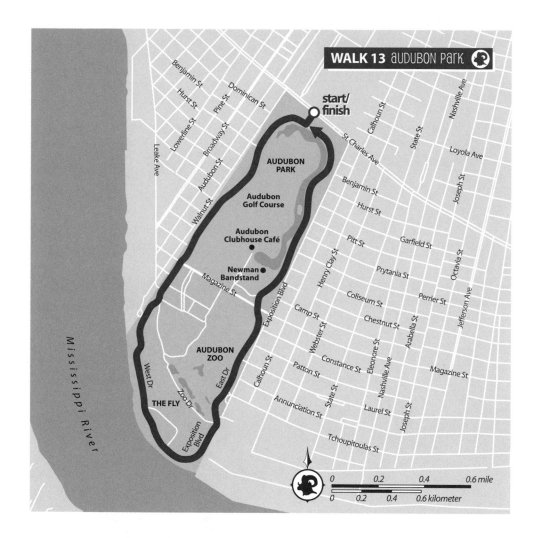

start/
finish

Benjamin St

Hurst St

Dominican St

Pine St

Lowerline St

Broadway St

Leake Ave

Audubon St

Walnut St

**AUDUBON
PARK**

St. Charles Ave

Calhoun St

Nashville Ave

State St

Loyola Ave

Benjamin St

Hurst St

Joseph St

**Audubon
Golf Course**

**Audubon
Clubhouse Café** •

Pitt St

Garfield St

Octavia St

Newman •
Bandstand

Henry Clay St

Prytania St

Perrier St

Jefferson Ave

Magazine St

Exposition Blvd

Coliseum St

Camp St

Webster St

Chestnut St

Eleonore St

Arabella St

**AUDUBON
ZOO**

West Dr

Zoo Dr

East Dr

Calhoun St

Constance St

Patton St

Nashville Ave

Magazine St

THE FLY

State St

Annunciation St

Laurel St

Joseph St

Exposition
Blvd

Tchoupitoulas St

Mississippi River

0   0.2   0.4   0.6 mile

0   0.2   0.4   0.6 kilometer

13 AUDUBON PARK: UPTOWN OASIS

BOUNDARIES: St. Charles Ave., Exposition Blvd., Mississippi River, Walnut St.
DISTANCE: 1.8 miles–3.2 miles (two options)
PARKING: Free parking along St. Charles Ave.; 2-hour parking in neighborhood
PUBLIC TRANSIT: St. Charles Ave. Streetcar

The folks at the Audubon Institute call Audubon Park an "urban oasis," and they couldn't have come up with a more appropriate description. With its duck-filled lagoon, ancient live oaks, and serene sitting areas, Audubon offers a respite to anyone looking to escape the pressures of life.

In historic Uptown New Orleans across from Tulane University, Audubon Park has a rich and fascinating history, having once been home to Native Americans and, many years later, the nation's first commercial sugarcane plantation. During the Civil War, the site alternately hosted a Confederate camp and a Union hospital.

The city acquired the land in 1871 for the purpose of hosting The World's Industrial and Cotton Centennial Exposition of 1884, Louisiana's first world's fair. At the time, the park was called Upper City Park, but city planners renamed it Audubon Park in 1886 in honor of artist-naturalist John James Audubon, who painted many of his iconic *Birds of America* in Louisiana.

With its development handed over to landscape architect John Charles Olmsted—whose family's firm designed New York's Central Park—Audubon became a full-fledged city park. Today, the 300-acre recreational area includes a 1.8-mile jogging trail, a 2.2-mile dirt path, a golf course, riding stables, picnic shelters, playgrounds, tennis courts, and soccer fields.

Local celebrities such as New Orleans Saints quarterback Drew Brees and political strategist James Carville, both of whom live in the neighborhood, are regular visitors to Audubon Park. And with the city's exploding film industry, other stars—Harrison Ford and Woody Harrelson among them—have been known to partake of the park's amenities.

- Begin at the front entrance of Audubon Park, on St. Charles Ave. across from Tulane University. Spend some time in the circular garden. Its fountains, sculpture, and vast array of blooms make this one of the park's most enticing stops.

- Continue onto the paved jogging trail in front of *The Travelers,* three sculptures by artist Deborah Masters. The trail is divided into a section for bikers and another for walkers and joggers. Be sure to stay on the correct side, and if you bring your dog, remember that leashes are mandatory.

- Turn right (west) at the sculptures and begin walking along the park's duck-filled lagoon. You're likely to see ducks, swans, and geese meandering along the shore, their honks and quacks mingling with the rumble of St. Charles Avenue streetcars. Visitors are welcome to bring stale bread to feed to them.

- Continue walking west along the trail. Even on the most sweltering of days, Audubon's ancient live oak trees provide enough shade to make walking bearable. Take some time to marvel at these spectacular moss-draped wonders of nature—they make Audubon so special.

- As you circle the trail and head south, you'll see the mansions of Walnut Street to your right and Cecile's Crepe Myrtle Grove to your left. One of many wedding venues in the park, the grove features gazebos at each end, a circular path, an open field, and dozens of crepe myrtle trees, whose pink and red blooms are at their peak in the summer. The area was dedicated to Cecile Usdin, a park patron who considered this her favorite spot on the park grounds.

- As you continue walking south, you'll notice the park's 18-hole golf course. Redesigned in 2001, the course features contoured Bermuda fairways, manicured Tif-Eagle greens, four lagoons, and exquisite landscaping. Entry is limited to those who are playing, but the Audubon Clubhouse Café, inside the clubhouse, is open to the public. Grab a table on the wraparound veranda and enjoy the view.

- As you approach Magazine Street, you may take one of two routes—continuing around the jogging trail or crossing Magazine Street and heading to the Riverview. This will add 1.4 miles to the walk but will take you right up to the banks of the Mississippi River.

- If you prefer to stay on the trail, continue walking on the trail past the rear entrance of the park; if you want to check out the Riverview, cross Magazine at West Drive. Note that Magazine is a heavily traveled roadway, so be extra-careful as you make your way across. Continue walking south. The buildings to your right are luxury condominiums. To your left is the award-winning Audubon Zoo, which, like the park itself, is part of the Audubon Institute's conglomeration of nature attractions. With its vast array of exotic animals, the zoo is well worth a separate visit.

- Around the 1-mile point, you'll have to cross a railroad track to get to the south side of the park. The Riverview is commonly known as The Fly, a reference to a butterfly-shaped river-viewing shelter built in the 1960s and demolished in the 1980s. The area is an ideal spot for picnicking, kite-flying, Frisbee-tossing, or relaxing with a good book. Benches line the riverfront, giving visitors an up-close view of barges and ships traveling to and from the Port of New Orleans.

- Make your way around The Fly, past the soccer and baseball fields, and turn north onto Exposition Boulevard, which will take you to the southeast corner of the park, past the tennis courts. Exposition eventually turns into East Drive, where one of the first sites you'll see on the left (near Annunciation Street) is the magnificent Tree of Life, one of the park's oldest trees and another popular wedding venue. Although no signs identify the tree, its massive roots and limbs, many of which droop to the ground, make it difficult to miss. Stop at the tree and take in its beauty before continuing down the roadway to The Labyrinth, a meditative space with a formal entry arch, walking trail, and benches. Adjacent to the The Labyrinth are the Cascade

The Gumbel Memorial Fountain, at the entrance of the park, is the work of Austrian sculptor Isidore Konti.

Stables, a state-of-the-art riding facility that offers lessons, show training, and 2-mile guided rides around the park.

- Cross Magazine St. and return to the north side of the park. Get back on the jogging trail and continue walking north. On the left, you'll see the Newman Bandstand, the only location in the park where amplified music is allowed. In that same area is the Louisiana Roll of Honor, a World War I memorial.

- Continue walking north past the stately homes of Exposition Boulevard to your right and—about halfway between Magazine and St. Charles—Bird Island, which has been part of Audubon Park for more than a century. The natural bird habitat is home to egrets, herons, and other wading birds.

- Continue walking north toward St. Charles Avenue. As you get closer, you'll see the tower of the Holy Name of Jesus Church and hear the rumbling of streetcars. Turn northwest and return to the front entryway.

POINTS OF INTEREST

Audubon Park and Audubon Zoo auduboninstitute.org, 6500 Magazine St., 504-581-4629

Audubon Golf Course auduboninstitute.org/visit/golf, 6500 Magazine St., 504-861-2537

Audubon Clubhouse Café auduboninstitute.org/visit/clubhouse-cafe, 6500 Magazine St., 504-212-5282

The Fly auduboninstitute.org/audubon-park/favorites/the-riverview, 504-861-2537

route summary

1. Enter park at St. Charles Avenue entrance.

2. Get on jogging trail a few feet away and walk west.

3. Circle around trail past mansions and golf course.

4. Walk south toward Magazine Street.

5. Cross Magazine at West Drive.

6. Walk along West, cross railroad track, and take path to river.

7. Walk on West along the riverfront to Exposition Boulevard.

8. Turn north at Exposition, which eventually turns into East Drive.

9. Take East back to Magazine.

10. Cross Magazine and return to north side of the park.

11. Get back on jogging trail and head north toward St. Charles.

12. Circle northwest at St. Charles and walk to park entrance.

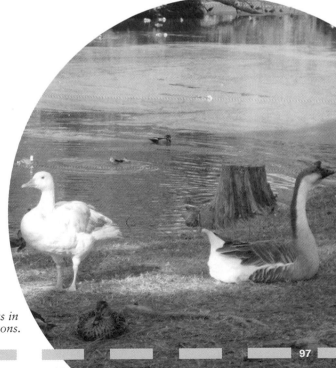

Ducks, swans, and other birds are common sights in and along Audubon Park's lagoons.

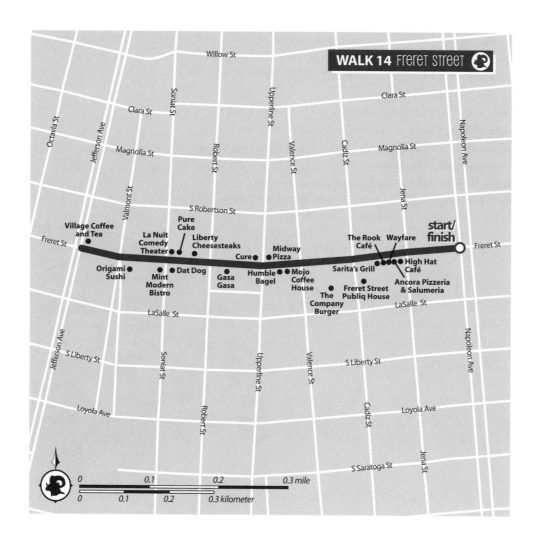

WALK 14 Freret Street

Willow St

Clara St

Soniat St

Upperline St

Clara St

Octavia Ave

Jefferson Ave

Magnolia St

Robert St

Valence St

Cadiz St

Magnolia St

Napoleon Ave

Valmont St

S Robertson St

Jena St

Village Coffee
and Tea

Freret St

Pure
Cake

La Nuit
Comedy
Theater

Liberty
Cheesesteaks

Cure

Midway
Pizza

The Rook
Café

Wayfare

start/
finish

Freret St

Origami
Sushi

Dat Dog

Gasa
Gasa

Humble
Bagel

Mojo
Coffee
House

Sarita's Grill

High Hat
Café

Mint
Modern
Bistro

The
Company
Burger

Freret Street
Publiq House

Ancora Pizzeria
& Salumeria

LaSalle St

LaSalle St

Jefferson Ave

S Liberty St

Soniat St

Upperline St

Valence St

S Liberty St

Napoleon Ave

Loyola Ave

Robert St

Cadiz St

Loyola Ave

S Saratoga St

Jena St

0   0.1   0.2   0.3 mile
0   0.1   0.2   0.3 kilometer

14 FrereT STreeT: FeeDING FreNZY

BOUNDARIES: **Freret St., Jefferson Ave., Napoleon Ave.**
PARKING: **Free lot at Freret and Jena Sts., free street parking**
PUBLIC TRANSIT: **RTA Bus #15 (Freret)**

It's no secret that New Orleans is one of the world's preeminent dining destinations, with some of the finest restaurants to be found in the French Quarter, the Warehouse District, and along Magazine Street. Now you can add Freret Street, between Jefferson and Napoleon Avenues, to the culinary mix.

Freret Street, named after the 19th-century mayor William Freret, is a haven for foodies. You won't find any fine-dining eateries on this eight-block stretch, but what you will discover are places specializing in fun and creative fare—gourmet hot dogs, for instance, and craft cocktails, along with po'boys, meat pies, doughnuts, and even a Louisiana take on the Philly cheesesteak. The growing number of businesses is equally impressive: salons, a comic book store, an art gallery, a garden center, and a secondhand-clothing shop, among others.

The transformation of Freret from nearly dead to alive and kicking is nothing short of a miracle. Though the street had been a thriving commercial strip in the mid-20th century, suburban sprawl and the murder of Bill Long, a beloved Freret Street baker, in the 1980s left the strip decayed and depressed.

Enter the Freret Business and Property Owner Association, a group of citizens that vowed "to establish an image that Freret Street is a safe, vibrant, easily accessible destination to shop, dine, play, work and live." They succeeded beyond anyone's imagination, and the growth of Freret continues to this day, with even more restaurants and businesses in the works.

● **Begin your walk at the corner of Napoleon Avenue and Freret Street in front of Holy Rosary Academy and High School, a Catholic school that opened in 1908 with 42 students. The building is the former home of Our Lady of Lourdes Church, which closed in 2008 as part of an Archdiocese of New Orleans reorganization. Across the street is a parking lot that is transformed into the Freret Market on the first Saturday**

cure

Neal Bodenheimer, a mixologist, was among the first proprietors to take his chances on Freret Street in 2009, and his decision to open the craft-cocktail bar Cure in an old firehouse inspired other business owners to follow suit.

Today, Freret is a thriving culinary corridor, with Cure one of its most popular destinations. Since opening, Cure has been named to *Esquire*'s list of Best Bars in America, *Travel & Leisure*'s list of America's Best Cocktail Bars, and *Food & Wine*'s Best Cocktail Bars in the US.

It's easy to see why. The menu features a fascinating collection of libations, including a tequila drink called the Mexican Bus Ride, a gin-based drink called Sleepless Again, and a Cognac creation called Dark in the Corner. Beer and wine selections are equally impressive.

"This classy bar has perfected the delicate act behind the perfectly balanced cocktail," *Travel & Leisure* wrote of Cure. "With a tremendous selection of spirits, a variety of house-made bitters, and a talented crew with a freakish bent for creativity, cocktails here never disappoint."

No need to starve at Cure either. The menu includes a variety of cheese trays; small plates such as steak tartare and maitake mushrooms; and a sandwich concoction called the Curewich, which combines fried eggs, Cheddar cheese, and braised bacon on a Weiss Guys roll.

of every month (except July and August). The market features art and produce vendors, live music, a children's area, and restaurants serving up their specialties.

● Walk one block to Jena Street. A little advice before you continue: Make sure you're hungry, and unless you know exactly where you want to dine, snack, or drink (maybe all three), browse a few menus so you have a feel for the variety of fare being served. Of course, nothing says you can't try something at every stop, right?

● On the corner of Jena and Freret is High Hat Café, located in the building that once housed Bill Long's Bakery and Deli. High Hat is known for its Southern cuisine, and among its specialties are fried catfish, barbecue shrimp, pimento cheese, and heavenly sides like pimento mac and cheese, stone-ground grits, and braised greens. Next door, Ancora's menu features Neopolitan pizza and house-made salumi.

- Wayfare, at 4510 Freret, specializes in the art of sandwich making, from The Knuckle (chilled roast beef, pickled red onion, shoestring potato crisps, horseradish aioli, and arugula on a pretzel bun) to the BL(fg)T (fried green tomato, Kurobuta bacon, shaved red onion, green leaf lettuce, arugula, spicy mayo, and sweet potato–habanero hot sauce on seven-grain bread). Just next door to Wayfare are The Rook Café, a coffee-house geared to tabletop-gaming fans; Sarita's Grill, a Latin-fusion café and one of the first businesses to open on the so-called New Freret; and the Freret Street Publiq House, a music club in an old supermarket.

- Cross Cadiz Street and you'll be in front of The Company Burger, one of the first of a proliferation of gourmet burger restaurants to open in New Orleans over the past five years. In 2013, the website Thrillist named its burgers among the top 33 in the United States. Its speciality is simple: twin patties, two slices of American cheese, house-made bread-and-butter pickles, and red onions.

- Continue walking down Freret and cross Valence Street. Bagel shops have come and gone in New Orleans, but Humble Bagel, at 4716 Freret St., seems to be filling a demand for the real deal, with kettle-boiled bagels like those found in America's best bagel shops. At the corner is Mojo Coffee House, a Wi-Fi café offering breakfast and lunch.

- Cross Upperline Street. In this block, you'll find Gasa Gasa (Japanese for "easily distracted"), one of the newest music venues in town, boasting a regular lineup of local bands and performers, along with art exhibitions, film screenings, and record-ing sessions.

Cross Robert Street and, at the end of the block, enjoy the colorful, funky scene that is Dat Dog, a hot dog joint that began in a 465-square-foot shed before moving to bigger digs—an old service station—across the street. That was back in 2011, and the place continues to grow in popularity with a second location on Magazine Street and a third on Frenchmen Street in the Marigny. The menu includes such dogs as alligator sausage, spicy chipotle veggie, and turducken (a trio of duck, turkey, and chicken). Even the fries are worth the splurge, especially the White Trash Fries, topped with chili, sour cream, guacamole, onions, cheese, and jalapenos. In 2013, Zagat named Dat Dog to its Top 10 list of Franks Worth Traveling For.

- Continue down Freret past two more restaurants—Mint, a Vietnamese bistro and bar, and Origami Sushi (because what's a culinary corridor without sushi?). Walk two more blocks and cross Freret at Jefferson Avenue, the halfway point of the Freret food crawl. Village Coffee offers a nice selection of pastries, salads, sandwiches, and coffee drinks, and its free Wi-Fi makes it an ideal study hall for students from nearby Tulane and Loyola Universities.

- Walk two blocks to the 5000 block of Freret. At the corner is La Nuit Comedy Theatre, which stages a variety of shows featuring some of the city's best comic talent. The club also offers improvisation, sketch writing, and children's acting classes. Also in this block is Pure Cake, which since opening in 2012 has won raves for its wedding cakes, mini-cakes, and cake pops, including flavors such as praline and bananas Foster. At Liberty Cheesesteak, the owners—including a native Philadelphian—serve up authentic Philly cheesesteaks (with onions and Cheez Whiz). Variations include a Cajun Chick Steak and a Steak Hoagie.

- Cross Robert Street. At the end of the block is Cure, the craft-cocktail bar whose owners get much of the credit for the Freret Street revival (see sidebar).

- As you make your way back to Napoleon, you'll pass three more restaurants: Midway Pizza, known for its deep-dish pie; Beaucoup Juice, where you can get fresh-juice snow balls, veggie juices, and smoothies with such names as Mardi Gras Mango, Chuck Berry, and The Tipitina (a mixture of strawberries, peaches, bananas, honey, and soy milk); and Freret Street Po-Boy and Donut Shop, whose signature items are actually fried-seafood platters and Creole red beans and rice.

POINTS OF INTEREST

High Hat Café highhatcafe.com, 4500 Freret St., 504-754-1336

Ancora Pizzeria & Salumeria ancorapizza.com, 4508 Freret, 504-324-1636

Wayfare wayfarenola.com, 4510 Freret St., 504-309-4510

The Rook Café facebook.com/therookcafe, 4516 Freret St., 618-520-9843

Sarita's Grill 4520 Freret St., 504-324-3562

Freret Street Publiq House publiqhouse.com, 4528 Freret St., 504-826-9912

The Company Burger thecompanyburger.com, 4600 Freret St., 504-267-0320

Mojo Coffee House facebook.com/mojofreret, 4700 Freret St., 504-875-2243

Humble Bagel humblebagel.com, 4716 Freret St., 504-355-3535

Gasa Gasa gasagasa.com, 4920 Freret St., Twitter: @gasagasanola

Dat Dog datdognola.com, 5030 Freret St., 504-899-6883

Mint Modern Bistro & Bar mintmodernbistro.com, 5100 Freret St., 504-218-5534

Origami Sushi sushinola.com, 5130 Freret St., 504-899-6532

Village Coffee and Tea villagecoffeenola.com, 5335 Freret St., 504-861-1909

La Nuit Comedy Theater nolacomedy.com, 5039 Freret St., 504-231-7011

Pure Cake purecakenola.com, 5035 Freret St., 504-872-0065

Liberty Cheesesteaks libertycheesesteaks.com, 5031 Freret St.,
504-875-4447

Cure curenola.com, 4905 Freret St., 504-302-2357

Midway Pizza midwaypizzanola.com, 4725 Freret St.,
504-322-2815

Beaucoup Juice facebook.com/beaucoupjuice,
4719 Freret St., 504-430-5508

Freret Street Po-Boy and Donut Shop
freretstreetpoboys.com, 4701 Freret St.,
504-872-9676

route summary

1.   Begin walk on Freret Street at Napoleon
     Avenue in front of Holy Rosary Academy.
2.   Walk eight blocks to Jefferson Avenue and
     cross Freret.
3.   Walk eight blocks back on Freret to Napoleon.

*Freret Street Publiq House is housed in what was
once a Canal Villere supermarket.*

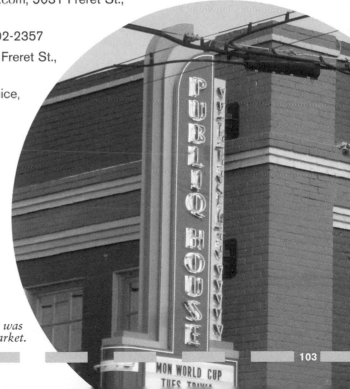

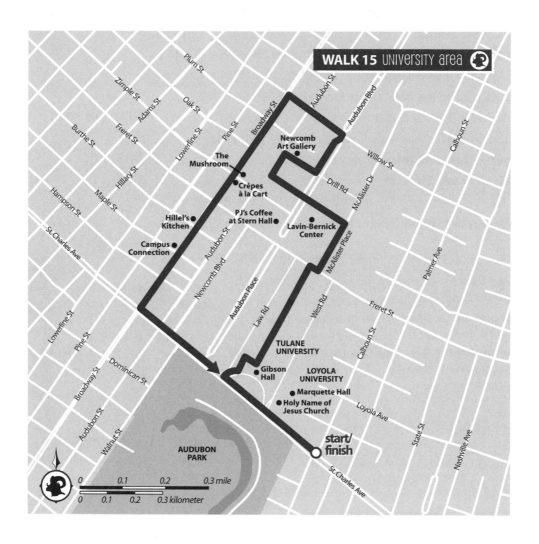

Plum St

Zimple St

Oak St

Adams St

Broadway St

Audubon St

Audubon Blvd

Calhoun St

Burthe St

Freret St

Pine St

Lowerline St

Newcomb Art Gallery

Willow St

The Mushroom

Crêpes à la Cart

Drill Rd

McAlister Dr

Hampson St

Hillary St

Maple St

Hillel's Kitchen

PJ's Coffee at Stern Hall

Lavin-Bernick Center

St Charles Ave

Campus Connection

Audubon Blvd

Newcomb Blvd

McAlister Place

Palmer Ave

Lowerline St

Pine St

Audubon Place

Law Rd

West Rd

Freret St

Calhoun St

TULANE UNIVERSITY

Broadway St

Dominican St

Gibson Hall

LOYOLA UNIVERSITY

Marquette Hall

Holy Name of Jesus Church

Loyola Ave

State St

Nashville Ave

Audubon St

Walnut St

AUDUBON PARK

start/ finish

St Charles Ave

0   0.1   0.2   0.3 mile

0   0.1   0.2   0.3 kilometer

15 UNIVERSITY area: academia amid the oaks

BOUNDARIES: St. Charles Ave., Calhoun St., Willow St., Broadway St.
DISTANCE: 2.3 miles
PARKING: Free parking on St. Charles, free 2-hour residential parking in neighborhood
PUBLIC TRANSIT: St. Charles Ave. Streetcar

New Orleans is home to myriad colleges and universities, but none are as stunning as the campuses of Tulane and Loyola Universities, which front historic St. Charles Avenue across from Audubon Park in a neighborhood of stately, jaw-dropping mansions.

Chartered in 1912, Loyola University New Orleans is one of 28 Jesuit colleges and universities in the United States. Spread out over 24 acres, it boasts an 11:1 student ratio and five colleges: business, humanities and natural sciences, law, music and fine arts, and social sciences.

Tulane, one of the nation's preeminent research universities, was founded as the Medical College of Louisiana in 1834, eventually merging with the public University of Louisiana. It debuted as the private Tulane University in 1884 when benefactor Paul Tulane, a wealthy merchant, donated more than $1 million in land, cash, and securities "for the promotion and encouragement of intellectual, moral, and industrial education." Tulane's academic divisions include architecture, social work, business, science and engineering, medicine, law, liberal arts, and public health and tropical medicine. In the fall of 2014, Tulane unveiled its newest gem: Yulman Stadium, bringing Green Wave football back to campus after a 40-year absence.

Tulane and Loyola enjoy a harmonious relationship. The two schools host many joint programs, and students with meal plans can dine at either campus.

● **Start at the north corner of St. Charles at Calhoun Street. Loyola's Communications/ Music Complex is to the right. The 115,000-square-foot structure is one of Loyola's newer, more modern buildings. It houses the College of Music and Fine Arts, the School of Mass Communication, and the Louis J. Roussel Performance Hall, Loyola's largest performance venue.**

- Continue down St. Charles Avenue past Marquette Hall, the oldest building on campus. Listed on the National Register of Historic Places, Marquette houses the office of Loyola's president as well as other administrative offices.

  Next to Marquette is the iconic Holy Name of Jesus Church, one of the city's most spectacular Catholic churches and home to such Loyola events as baccalaureate ceremonies, choral concerts, and school-year-opening Mass. The church was founded in 1886. Stained glass with various memorials adorns the upper windows.

- Cross West Road and continue down St. Charles past Gibson Hall, Tulane's main administrative building. The oldest building on Tulane's Uptown campus, Gibson was built in 1894 in the Richardsonian Romanesque style of stone over brick. It houses the admissions office and the offices of the university president, provost, and other senior-level executives. The TULANE UNIVERSITY sign in front of Gibson is one of the most photographed spots on campus.

- Turn right onto campus just before Law Road. The building to the left is Tilton Hall, home to the Amistad Research Center, a manuscripts library for the study of ethnic history and culture and race relations in the United States. Built in 1902, the building also houses the Murphy Institute of Political Economy, which supports research in public policy, public affairs, and civic engagement and seeks to educate students on the most challenging of economic, moral, and political problems.

- Turn right between Tilton and Dinwiddie Halls, past the rear side of Gibson. At the center stairway of Gibson, turn left and walk through the Academic Quad. As you walk through the Quad, marvel at the spectacular live oak trees and, if it's springtime, garden upon garden of hot-pink azaleas. In 2013, Tulane was named to BuzzFeed's list of 41 Scenic College Campuses That Were Made for Instagram, and its lushness and architecturally historic buildings are certainly two reasons why.

  To the right is the Richardson Memorial Building, which houses Tulane's acclaimed School of Architecture. In front of the school is the famous Mardi Gras bead tree, where strands of colorful plastic beads hang like moss. During Carnival season, students enjoy gathering at the tree and adding to its decor.

- As you walk through the Quad, keep an eye out for several pieces of outdoor sculpture. Among them are *Timber,* a structure made of glass, steel, and wood by Gene Koss, and *Arcs in Disorder,* one of the trademark works of French artist Bernar Venet.

- Continue walking down the middle walkway past Cudd Hall and the old School of Social Work building to the left and Stanley Thomas Hall to the right. You are now in Tulane's science-and-engineering hub, where in addition to the traditional sciences, students can choose from such majors as biomedical engineering, evolutionary biology, and computer science. One of the newest buildings on campus is the Donna and Paul Flower Hall for Research and Innovation, a contemporary four-story building set behind a towering oak. With its cutting-edge labs, Flower serves as a vital part of the city's growing bioscience and chemical-engineering sectors.

- Just ahead is PJ's Coffee, where you can stop for an iced latte, mocha, or lemonade—that is, unless students are between classes. That's when the café is at its busiest, with professors and students grabbing cups of joe en route to their next class.

- Cross Freret Street, one of the major streets that runs through campus, and continue straight onto McAlister Place, a landscaped pedestrian mall and popular gathering spot. In the fall of 2013, actors Channing Tatum and Jonah Hill filmed parts of *22 Jump Street* along the walkway, attracting hundreds of giddy, photo-snapping students—all on their way to class.

To the right is Devlin Fieldhouse, home of Tulane's men's and women's basketball teams. Just past Devlin is the Lavin-Bernick Center for University Life, also known as the LBC. The LBC is home to the bookstore, dining venues, conference rooms, study lounges, and outdoor patios, including one that overlooks the LBC Quad. On Friday afternoons, students begin the weekend with "Fridays on the Quad," a party featuring bands, food trucks, inflatables, and other activities.

Across from the LBC are the ultramodern Goldring/Woldenberg Halls I and II, home of the A. B. Freeman School of Business. Next door is McAlister Auditorium, which boasts the world's largest self-suspended concrete dome. The auditorium is used for concerts and lectures. In the fall of 2014, a scene from the upcoming film *Our Brand Is Crisis,* produced by George Clooney and starring Sandra Bullock, was shot here.

- Turn left in front of the LBC and walk a block to Newcomb Place. Cross Newcomb and enter the Newcomb Quad, once the home of H. Sophie Newcomb Memorial College, the first women's coordinate college within a US university. Walk around the Quad, beginning with Dixon Hall to your left. Dixon is one of the city's most popular performance venues and home to the acclaimed Summer Lyric Theatre. Other buildings on this part of campus include Newcomb Hall, the architectural centerpiece of Newcomb College; Woldenberg Art Center, home to the Newcomb Art Gallery, which is free and open to the public; and Dixon Hall Annex, where the New Orleans Shakespeare Festival at Tulane and other performance ensembles are based.

- Circle around the Quad and turn left at Newcomb Place. Walk a block past the Caroline Richardson Building and the University Health Center to Willow Street. Turn left on Willow and walk two blocks to Broadway Street. Though not part of Tulane's campus, Broadway is the center of Greek life at Tulane, with many of the homes occupied by fraternities and sororities.

- Walk one block to Zimple Street. The high-rise to your left is Tulane's newest residence hall—the Barbara Greenbaum House at Newcomb Lawn. Continue down Broadway past a strip of commericial establishments, including the Mushroom record store and Crêpes à la Cart.

  The large yellow building at the corner of Broadway and Burthe is home to Tulane Hillel, which serves Tulane's significant Jewish student community. Hillel's Kitchen is a fully kosher restaurant open to the public, with menu items such as matzah ball soup, falafel, and bagels.

- Continue walking south on Broadway toward St. Charles Avenue. Campus Connection, at the corner of Maple Street, stocks an array of Greek merchandise as well as a wide variety of Tulane T-shirts, sweatshirts, and hats.

- At St. Charles, turn left and walk to Audubon Place, one of the Crescent City's most exclusive neighborhoods. Audubon Place is private, so you'll only be able to catch a glimpse from outside the gates. Do take note of #2 Audubon Place, the white-pillared mansion that fronts St. Charles. Built in 1907, the Georgian Revival house was the home of United Fruit Company magnate Samuel Zemurray for decades before he donated it to Tulane to serve as the official residence of the university president.

- Cross Audubon Place and continue walking past Gibson Hall back the starting point.

POINTS OF INTEREST

Loyola University New Orleans loyno.edu, 6363 St. Charles Ave., 504-865-3240

Holy Name of Jesus Church hnjchurch.org, 6367 St. Charles Ave., 504-865-7430

Tulane University tulane.edu, 6823 St. Charles Ave., 504-865-5000

PJ's Coffee at Stern Hall pjscoffee.com, 7001 Freret St., 504-865-5705

Lavin-Bernick Center tulane.edu/studentaffairs/lbc, McAlister Place, 504-865-5705

Newcomb Art Gallery newcombartgallery.tulane.edu, Newcomb Quad, 504-865-5328

Crêpes à la Cart crepecaterer.com, 1039 Broadway St., 504-866-2362

The Mushroom facebook.com/mushroomnola, 1037 Broadway St., 504-866-6065

Hillel's Kitchen hknola.com, 912 Broadway St., 504-909-9919

Campus Connection campusconnection.cc, 800 Broadway St., 504-866-8552

route summary

1. Begin walk at St. Charles Avenue and Calhoun Street.
2. Walk two blocks and turn right onto campus just before Law Road.
3. Walk past Gibson Hall (main administration building) and turn right onto walkway.
4. Walk down Gibson Quad to Freret Street.
5. Cross Freret and continue on McAlister Place.
6. Walk down McAlister and turn left in front of Lavin-Bernick Center.
7. Walk to Newcomb Place and enter Newcomb Quad.
8. Circle around Newcomb Quad and turn left on Newcomb Place.
9. Walk to Willow Street, turn left, and walk to Broadway Street.
10. Cross Broadway and turn left.
11. Walk down St. Charles back to the starting point.

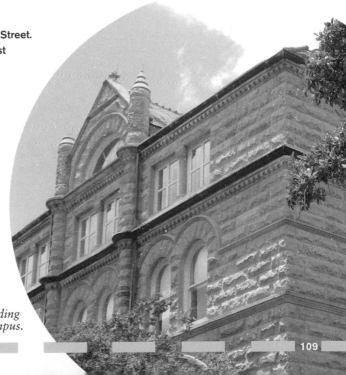

Built in 1894, Gibson Hall is the oldest building on the Tulane campus.

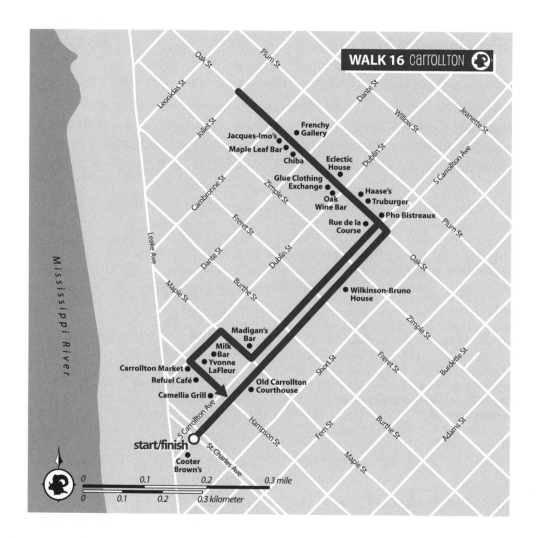

WALK 16 carrollton

Mississippi River

Oak St

Plum St

Leonidas St

Joliet St

Dante St

Willow St

Jeanette St

Frenchy Gallery

Jacques-Imo's

Maple Leaf Bar

Chiba

Eclectic House

Dublin St

S Carrollton Ave

Glue Clothing Exchange

Cambronne St

Zimple St

Oak Wine Bar

Haase's

Truburger

Pho Bistreaux

Plum St

Freret St

Rue de la Course

Dante St

Dublin St

Oak St

Leake Ave

Maple St

Burthe St

Wilkinson-Bruno House

Zimple St

Burdette St

Madigan's Bar

Milk Bar

Yvonne LaFleur

Short St

Freret St

Carrollton Market

Refuel Café

Old Carrollton Courthouse

Camellia Grill

S Carrollton Ave

start/finish

Cooter Brown's

St. Charles Ave

Hampson St

Fern St

Burthe St

Maple St

Adams St

0   0.1   0.2   0.3 mile

0   0.1   0.2   0.3 kilometer

16 Carrollton: Old-Time Charm with Funky Feel

BOUNDARIES: St. Charles Ave., S. Carrollton Ave., Oak St., Dublin St.
DISTANCE: 1.54 miles
PARKING: Free parking on St. Charles, metered parking on Carrollton
PUBLIC TRANSIT: St. Charles Ave. Streetcar

The Carrollton neighborhood has a rich and fascinating history dating back to the mid-18th century, when, as the town of Carrollton, it was the seat of Jefferson Parish. Carrollton was annexed by New Orleans in 1874, but remnants of the old days remain—including the pillared structure that once housed the town's courthouse but which has been home to several schools ever since.

With its majestic oak trees, streetcar line, and quaint commercial districts, the neighborhood still has a folksy, small-town feel. Yet in spite of its many transformations over the years, it is one of the city's most vibrant neighborhoods. Much of the credit goes to the revitalization of Oak Street, a funky street with old-time charm. On Oak, you'll find galleries, restaurants, cafés, secondhand stores, and the like. In 2010, *O, The Oprah Magazine* named the street as one of its "100 Things That Are (Actually) Getting Better."

These days, Oak Street is synonymous with po'boys, the ubiquitous sandwich that's as popular in New Orleans as cheesesteaks are in Philly. You won't find any famous po'boy shops on Oak (though you can get a heavenly roast beef at Jacques-Imo's), but every November, the street shuts down for the Oak Street Po-Boy Festival. With more than 30 vendors serving such po'boys as shrimp and crabmeat, barbecued oyster, drunken pig, and brisket with blue cheese, dieting—or maybe even fasting—the week before is highly advisable!

● Begin at the corner of St. Charles Avenue and South Carrollton Avenue in front of Cooter Brown's, a popular dive sports bar with an impressive oyster bar and beer selection. Cross St. Charles, but be extra-careful, as this is one of the area's busiest intersections.

● Continue two blocks on Carrollton to the stretch between Hampson and Maple Streets. Dating back to the 1850s, the building to your right once served as the courthouse for the town of Carrollton. It has also been home to several schools, including John McDonogh No. 23 School, Benjamin Franklin High School, and Lusher Extension School. Audubon Charter School vacated the building in May 2014, and the future of this historic structure was yet to be determined.

- **Cross Maple Street.** Though not included on this walk, Maple Street is certainly worth a side visit. Its boutiques, restaurants, cafés, and bars are especially popular with students from nearby Tulane and Loyola Universities.

- Continue down Carrollton past the Wilkinson-Bruno House, a Gothic Revival–style home built in 1846 and listed on the National Register of Historic Places. Adjacent to this house, between Oak and Zimple Streets, is St. Andrew's Episcopal Church. Cross Oak, turn left, cross Carrollton, and continue walking on the north side of Oak, in front of an old bank building that now houses a nail salon and Pho Bistreaux, a Vietnamese restaurant.

- Oak Street is like a small town unto itself where you can get your hair cut, your bike fixed, or your pet groomed. Oak extends all the way to the river, but this walk will take you five blocks to Joliet Street. Along the north side are Truburger, serving gourmet burgers and hot dogs; Haase's, a children's shoe and clothing store that has been in business for decades; Eclectic Home, an interiors shop; the Advocacy Center, a nonprofit group that offers legal services to seniors and people with disabilities; and Frenchy Gallery, whose owner, Frenchy, travels the country painting scenes from live performances such as sporting events and music festivals.

- Cross Oak at Joliet and continue along the south side of Oak. The two most popular venues on Oak—Jacques-Imo's and the Maple Leaf Bar—are situated side by side between Cambronne and Dante Streets. Do yourself a favor and plan a night around these two landmarks. Jacques-Imo's is a casual eatery that serves some of the tastiest food in town, from shrimp-and-alligator-sausage cheesecake to Godzilla Meets Fried Green Tomatoes (a soft-shell-crab dish). On any given night, the place is packed, and reservations are accepted only for parties of five or more. If you want a real dining adventure, consider reserving the colorful pickup truck that's parked in front. In the back of the truck is a table for two, the perfect spot for people-watching.

The Maple Leaf Bar is one of the city's most venerable music clubs, offering an array of music from jazz and blues to zydeco and funk. Among the club's regulars are the Rebirth Brass Band, funk and R&B musician Jon Cleary, and Bonerama. Over the years, unannounced sit-in guests have included the likes of Bruce Springsteen and Bonnie Raitt.

- Walk four blocks back to Carrollton Avenue, past even more restaurants, galleries, and shops. They include Chiba, an upscale sushi eatery; Oak Wine Bar, which also has live music; and Glue Clothing Exchange, a vintage-garment store. Grab a cup of java at Rue de la Course at the corner of Carrollton and Oak, which, like Pho Bistreaux across the street, is housed in an old bank building.

- Turn right at Carrollton and walk four blocks to Maple Street. Turn right at Maple in front of Madigan's Bar and continue walking in the heart of the Riverbend neighborhood. The strip shopping center on the left features one of the best sandwich and shake shops in town: The Milk Bar, where you can order such concoctions as Psycho Chicken, Cattle Fodder, and Wolf Me Down. Shakes include Mocha Madness, Butterscotch Hop, and Strawberry Fields.

- Cross Dublin Street, turn left, and walk a block to Hampson Street. In this neighborhood, you'll find almost every ethnic food imaginable—Indian at Taj of India, Spanish at Barcelona Tapas, and Japanese at Hana, among the choices. At the corner of Hampson and Dublin is Yvonne LaFleur, an upscale boutique known for its custom millinery, signature fragrances, and resplendent ball and wedding gowns. Also on Hampson are Refuel Café, a contemporary diner, and Carrollton Market, a modern Southern eatery and one of the latest hot spots to hit the New Orleans culinary scene.

- Turn right at Carrollton and continue walking past O'Henry's Food & Spirits, where you can throw the peanut shells on the floor, and the Camellia Grill, perhaps the most famous landmark in the whole neighborhood. The Grill, as locals call it, opened in 1946, and—except for a few years post-Katrina—has been serving up burgers, omelets, waffles, and other diner fare ever since. The food is good, but the waiters are better: They're funny, friendly, and full of spunk.

- Continue walking down Carrollton past the Shell service station, cross St. Charles Avenue, and return to the starting point—unless you want one last refreshment at New Orleans Original Daiquiris, to your right at 8100 St. Charles. Remember: In New Orleans, you can take your drinks to go.

POINTS OF INTEREST

Cooter Brown's cooterbrowns.com, 509 S. Carrollton Ave., 504-866-9104

Maple Street visitmaplestreet.com

Pho Bistreaux phobistreaux.biz, 1200 S. Carrollton Ave., 504-304-8334

Truburger truburgernola.com, 8115 Oak St., 504-218-5416

Haase's haases.com, 8119 Oak St., 504-866-9944

Eclectic Home eclectichome.net, 8211 Oak St., 504-866-6654

Frenchy Gallery frenchylive.com, 8319 Oak St., 504-861-7595

Jacques-Imo's jacques-imos.com, 8324 Oak St., 504-861-0886

Maple Leaf Bar mapleleafbar.com, 8316 Oak St., 504-866-9359

Chiba chiba-nola.com, 8312 Oak St., 504-826-9119

Glue Clothing Exchange glueclothingexchange.com, 8206 Oak St., 504-782-0619

Oak Wine Bar oaknola.com, 8118 Oak St., 504-302-1485

Rue de la Course facebook.com/ruedelacourse, 1140 S. Carrollton Ave., 504-861-4343

Madigan's Bar 800 S. Carrollton Ave., 504-866-9455

The Milk Bar 710 S. Carrollton Ave., 504-309-3310

Yvonne LaFleur yvonnelafleur.com, 8131 Hampson St., 504-866-9666

Carrollton Market carrolltonmarket.com, 8132 Hampson St., 504-252-9928

Refuel Café refuelcafe.com, 8124 Hampson St., 504-872-0187

O'Henry's Food & Spirits ohenrys.com, 632 Carrollton Ave., 504-866-9741

Camellia Grill 626 S. Carrollton Ave., 504-309-2679

route summary

1. Start at Cooter Brown's on South Carrollton Avenue.
2. Walk six blocks to Oak Street.
3. Turn left at Oak and cross Carrollton.
4. Walk four blocks to Joliet Street.
5. Cross Oak and turn left.
6. Walk four blocks back to Carrollton.
7. Turn right and walk four blocks to Maple Street.
8. Turn right and walk one block to Dublin Street.
9. Cross Dublin and turn left.
10. Walk one block to Hampson Street and turn left.
11. Walk one block to Carrollton and turn right.
12. Walk one block to starting point.

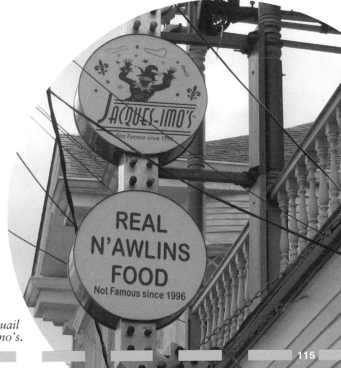

Fried grits, potato-crusted drum, and stuffed quail are among the tempting menu items at Jacques-Imo's.

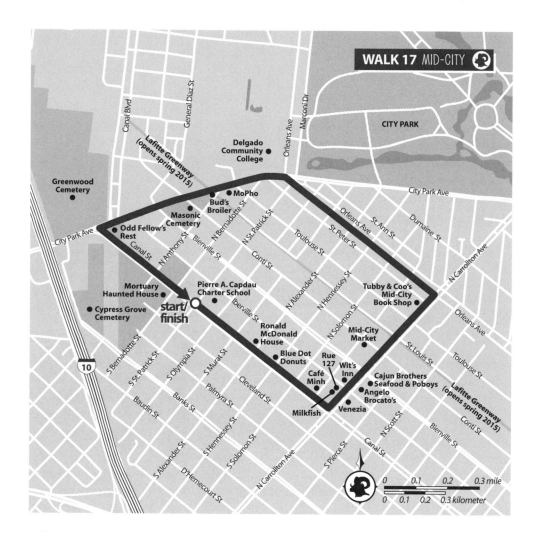

WALK 17 MID-CITY

CITY PARK

Greenwood Cemetery

Lafitte Greenway (opens spring 2015)

Delgado Community College

MoPho

Bud's Broiler

Masonic Cemetery

Odd Fellow's Rest

City Park Ave

City Park Ave

Orleans Ave

St. Ann St

Dumaine St

N Carrollton Ave

Orleans Ave

Canal St

N Anthony St

Bienville St

Conti St

Toulouse St

St. Peter St

N Bernadotte St

N St. Patrick St

N Alexander St

N Hennessey St

N Solomon St

Tubby & Coo's Mid-City Book Shop

Mortuary Haunted House

Pierre A. Capdau Charter School

start/ finish

Cypress Grove Cemetery

Iberville St

Ronald McDonald House

Mid-City Market

Blue Dot Donuts

Rue 127

Wit's Inn

Café Minh

Cajun Brothers Seafood & Poboys

Angelo Brocato's

St. Louis St

Toulouse St

Orleans Ave

Milkfish

Venezia

Lafitte Greenway (opens spring 2015)

Conti St

Bienville St

S Bernadotte St

S St. Patrick St

S Olympia St

S Murat St

Cleveland St

Palmyra St

Banks St

Baudin St

S Alexander St

S Hennessey St

S Solomon St

D'Hemecourt St

N Carrollton Ave

S Pierce St

Canal St

N Scott St

General Diaz St

Canal Blvd

Marconi Dr

0   0.1   0.2   0.3 mile

0   0.1   0.2   0.3 kilometer

MID-CITY: NEIGHBORHOOD REBIRTH

BOUNDARIES: **Canal St., N. Carrollton Ave., Orleans Ave., City Park Ave.**
DISTANCE: **2.4 miles**
PARKING: **Free on the street**
PUBLIC TRANSIT: **Canal Streetcar (Cemeteries and City Park/Museum Lines)**

Like so many neighborhoods in New Orleans, Mid-City was barely recognizable after Hurricane Katrina in 2005. Levee breaches caused extensive flooding to homes and businesses, leaving residents wondering whether their beloved community could survive the devastation.

Not only did it survive, it made one of the most successful comebacks of any New Orleans neighborhood, thanks to the spirit and will of its residents—and a whole slew of volunteers—whose determination to rebuild made it one of the most enviable parts of town.

As its name suggests, Mid-City is the true heart of New Orleans. Listed on the National Register of Historic Places, it consists mostly of structures built in the late 19th and early 20th centuries. The residential section largely consists of bungalows, Creole cottages, and shotguns—narrow homes with rooms arranged one behind the other. And while Mid-City has long had a bustling commercial zone, Katrina rebuilding has given the area a whole new energy and vibe, especially on North Carrollton Avenue between Canal Street and Orleans Avenue.

Of course, a New Orleans neighborhood wouldn't be complete without a festival, and one of the best is the Mid-City Bayou Boogaloo, another post-Katrina achievement. In fact, the festival began just a few months after Katrina to help revitalize the area and bring respite and joy to those struggling to rebuild. It has been growing in size and quality ever since.

● **Begin at Canal and North Saint Patrick Streets in front of Pierre A. Capdau Charter School, a K–8 school operated by New Beginnings Schools Foundation. Capdau opened in 2004 as one of the first charter schools in New Orleans. Today, all but a handful of city schools are charters, most having opened after Katrina, when educators saw the storm's devastation as an opportunity to rebuild New Orleans's long-troubled school system. Across Canal from Capdau is St. Anthony of Padua Catholic Church, one of dozens of churches of the Archdiocese of New Orleans.**

- Facing Canal Street, turn left and walk three blocks to North Alexander Street. The big yellow house on the corner is the Ronald McDonald House, which provides a "home away from home" for families with children suffering from cancer. Opened in 1983, it is one of nearly 340 such houses around the world. Among other things, the house offers comfortable beds, laundry and shower facilities, playrooms, and warm meals, most prepared by a dedicated corps of volunteers.

- Walk one block to North Hennessey Street. The bright-blue building you'll pass on your left is Blue Dot Donuts (4301 Canal), notable for being founded by three New Orleans police officers. Boasting more than 50 kinds of doughnuts, it's been featured on the Cooking Channel and the Food Network.

- Continue walking down Canal to North Carrollton Avenue. During this stretch, you'll pass Café Minh, an upscale Vietnamese restaurant, and across Canal, the local offices of Volunteers of America.

- Turn left at North Carrollton. If you're hungry or just in the mood for a drink, the next two blocks offer an array of choices. Among other ethnic cuisines, you'll find Italian, Chinese, Mexican, and Japanese. There's Milkfish, New Orleans's only Filipino restaurant; the upscale Rue 127, a New American bistro; Juicy Lucy's, for stuffed burgers; and Wit's Inn, a sports bar with some surprisingly good pizza. Brown Butter Southern Kitchen & Bar is the new kid on the block, and Venezia, across the street, is an old-school Italian restaurant that's been in business since 1957.

  Wherever you go, save room for dessert. Angelo Brocato's, with its homemade gelato, cannolis, and other Italian pastries, is a must. The old-fashioned ice-cream parlor is a replica of the one the Brocato family opened in Sicily in the early 20th century. At the corner of North Carrollton and Bienville is Cajun Brothers Seafood & Poboys, a seafood shop with some of the tastiest boiled crawfish in town. (Crawfish season runs from early March through the end of June.)

- Continue walking down North Carrollton. Between Bienville and St. Louis Streets is Mid-City Market, a commercial development that opened in 2013. The center, which consists largely of chains such as Panera Bread, Five Guys, and Pinkberry, replaced an old car dealership that had sat dormant and blighted since Katrina.

Adjacent to Mid-City Market, at St. Louis Street, is a segment of the Lafitte Greenway, a 2.6-mile multiuse trail and linear park. As of this writing, the greenway was still under construction but expected to open in the spring of 2015, connecting the French Quarter to Bayou St. John and Mid-City.

Two blocks down on North Carrollton, in a two-story Victorian house between Toulouse and St. Peter Streets, is Tubby & Coo's Mid-City Book Shop, which opened in late 2014 and specializes in such "nerdy" genres as sci-fi and fantasy (think Harry Potter, Dungeons and Dragons, and Doctor Who).

● Walk another four blocks to Orleans Avenue and turn left. Except for a school and a day-care center, this is a residential area known mostly for its Endymion parade celebrations. The Krewe of Endymion, with its dazzling double-decker floats, is one of the most spectacular parades of the Mardi Gras season, and throngs of revelers crowd the Orleans Avenue neutral ground in anticipation. The parade begins at Orleans and City Park Avenue and travels all the way to the Mercedes-Benz Superdome for the Endymion Extravaganza, a star-studded afterparty. But it's along this stretch of Orleans where the real partying takes place: The area is in such demand for parade viewing that many folks camp out days ahead of time to ensure they have a prime spot.

● From North Carrollton walk eight blocks to City Park Avenue. To the right is City Park (see the next walk), which at 1,300 acres is one of the largest urban parks in the United States. Across City Park Avenue is Delgado Community College, Louisiana's oldest and largest two-year college. Delgado offers 35 associate-degree programs, dozens of certificate and technical-diploma programs, and more than 100 noncredit courses. The largest programs include nursing, general studies, criminal justice, computer information technology, and culinary arts.

Across from Delgado is a commercial strip that includes MoPho, a Southeast Asian café whose chef, Michael Gulotta, once worked in the kitchen of Restaurant August, one of the Crescent City's top-rated restaurants. Pepper jelly–braised clams, crispy chicken wings, and pork-shoulder spring rolls are among its heavenly menu offerings.

● Continue walking down City Park Avenue; be extra-cautious, as parts of the sidewalk are broken up. At the corner of Toulouse Street is Bud's Broiler, a locally owned hamburger chain that's been around since the 1950s. Bud's is a true burger joint, with nothing to look at on the inside except a menu that gives the newer gourmet-burger places in town a run for their money. Try the burger with grated Cheddar and smoked hickory sauce, and be sure to add an order of onion rings and a chocolate milkshake.

● Just past Bud's, you'll be entering one of the largest collections of cemeteries in New Orleans. Often referred to as "cities of the dead" because of their aboveground grave sites, they include the Masonic, Cypress Grove, Greenwood, and St. Patrick's. Turn left at Canal Street and you'll encounter Odd Fellow's Rest, the Charity Hospital cemetery, and a Jewish cemetery. Each cemetery has its own fascinating background. Cypress Grove, for example, was the first cemetery built to honor the city's volunteer firefighters and their families. Odd Fellow's was built to provide a burial site for Protestant African Americans, who were barred from being buried with whites.

● As you head back to your starting point on North St. Patrick, take note of the Victorian mansion across Canal at the corner of St. Bernadotte Street. Built as a private residence in 1872 by Mary Slattery and renovated in subsequent years by various other owners, the mansion served as P. J. McMahon & Sons Funeral Home from 1930 to 1985. It is now used as a special-events venue and, come October, as the Mortuary Haunted House—known for being so spooky that those under 18 are discouraged from visiting. During the year, paranormal experts lead ghost tours and ghosthunting investigations, sharing "the secret legendary history of the mansion and why some of the souls that passed through the home never left."

POINTS OF INTEREST

Ronald McDonald House rmhc-nola.org, 4403 Canal St., 504-486-6668

Blue Dot Donuts bluedotdonuts.com, 4301 Canal St., 504-218-4866

Café Minh cafeminh.com, 4139 Canal St., 504-482-6266

Rue 127 rue127.com, 127 N. Carrollton Ave., 504-483-1571

Juicy Lucy's msjuicylucy.com, 133 N. Carrollton Ave., 504-598-5044

Wit's Inn witsinn.com, 141 N. Carrollton Ave., 504-486-1600

Brown Butter Southern Kitchen & Bar brownbutterrestaurant.com, 231 N. Carrollton Ave., 504-609-3871

Venezia venezianeworleans.net, 134 N. Carrollton Ave., 504-488-7991

Angelo Brocato's angelobrocatoicecream.com/aboutus.shtm, 214 N. Carrollton Ave., 504-486-1465

Cajun Brothers Seafood & Poboys facebook.com/cajunbrothersseafood, 236 N. Carrollton Ave., 504-488-7503

Mid-City Market mid-citymarket.com, 401 N. Carrollton Ave.

Lafitte Greenway (opens spring 2015) Basin Street to Canal Boulevard, folc-nola.org, 504-462-0645

Tubby & Coo's Mid-City Book Shop tubbyandcoos.com, 631 N. Carrollton Ave., 504-598-5536

City Park neworleanscitypark.com, 1 Palm Drive, 504-482-4888

MoPho mophonola.com, 514 City Park Ave., 504-482-6845

Bud's Broiler budsbroiler.com, 500 City Park Ave., 504-486-2559

Canal Street Cemeteries saveourcemeteries.org

Mortuary Haunted House hauntedmortuary.com, 4800 Canal St., 504-483-2350

route summary

1. Begin walk at Canal Street and North St. Patrick Street.
2. Walk seven blocks to North Carrollton Avenue and turn left.
3. Walk seven blocks to Orleans Avenue and turn left.
4. Walk eight blocks to City Park Avenue and turn left.
5. Walk six blocks to Canal Street and turn left.
6. Walk three blocks back to North St. Patrick, the starting point.

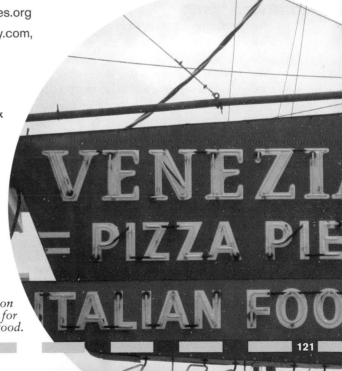

Despite increasing competition on North Carrollton, Venezia is the go-to spot for old-school Italian food.

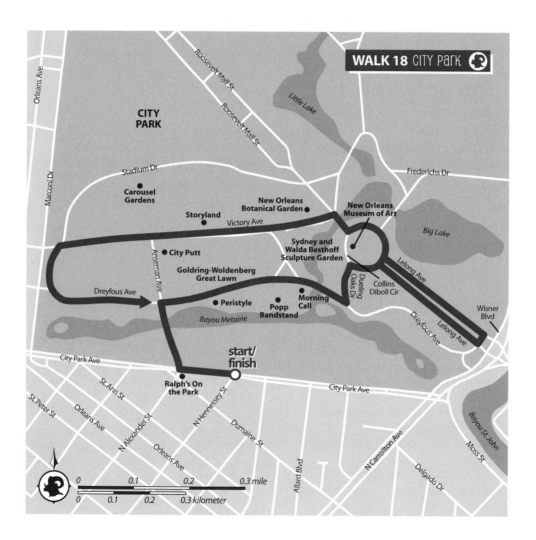

WALK 18 CITY PARK

CITY PARK

Little Lake

Orleans Ave

Marconi Dr

Roosevelt Mall St

Roosevelt Mall St

Stadium Dr

Frederichs Dr

Carousel Gardens

Storyland

New Orleans Botanical Garden

New Orleans Museum of Art

Big Lake

Victory Ave

City Putt

Sydney and Walda Besthoff Sculpture Garden

Anseman Ave

Goldring-Woldenberg Great Lawn

Lelong Ave

Dreyfous Ave

Peristyle

Popp Bandstand

Morning Call

Collins Diboll Cir

Dueling Oaks Dr

Bayou Metairie

Dreyfous Ave

Lelong Ave

Wisner Blvd

City Park Ave

start/ finish

Ralph's On the Park

City Park Ave

St. Peter St

St. Ann St

Orleans Ave

N Alexander St

N Hennessey St

Orleans Ave

Dumaine St

N Carrollton Ave

Allard Blvd

Delgado Dr

Bayou St. John

Moss St

0   0.1   0.2   0.3 mile

0   0.1   0.2   0.3 kilometer

18 CITY PARK: WONDERLAND OF FUN

BOUNDARIES: City Park Ave., Marconi Dr., Wisner Blvd., Victory Ave.
DISTANCE: 1.47 miles
PARKING: Free on the street or in the park
PUBLIC TRANSIT: Canal Streetcar (City Park/Museum Line)

City Park is a 1,300-acre wonderland—and Hurricane Katrina spared none of it. The 2005 storm and subsequent federal levee breaches flooded one of the country's largest and oldest urban parks, leaving sections of it with up to 8 feet of water and causing $43 million in damage.

Fast-forward nine years, and the park is better than ever, thanks to the dedication of volunteers from around the country and Friends of City Park, the park's fundraising arm. Back are most of the park's treasured staples, from the New Orleans Botanical Garden and Storyland to Carousel Gardens and the New Orleans Museum of Art, including the Sydney and Walda Besthoff Sculpture Garden. Its trees are as magnificent as ever, despite the park having lost 2,000 of them in the storm.

New attractions include City Putt, a 36-hole miniature golf course; the Goldring-Woldenberg Great Lawn, an expansive green space used for concerts and other activities; and the stunning Big Lake, with its surrounding bike and jogging paths.

In the coming years, the park will be home to a reimagined Louisiana Children's Museum (currently in the Warehouse District; see Walk 1), a splash park, and a new championship-level golf course.

If that weren't enough, the park is also home to two of the Crescent City's premier events: the Voodoo Music Experience in October and Celebration in the Oaks, one of the country's most spectacular holiday-lights festivals. Since 2008, City Park has also been the site of such movies and TV shows as *The Expendables, Now You See Me,* and *22 Jump Street.*

Bear in mind that this walk covers only a section of the park. Feel free to explore its other gems, such as the Popp Fountain, the disc-golf course, the new NOLA City Bark dog park, and the Couturie Forest and Arboretum, on your own. *Note:* Some roads in the park aren't

SYDNEY AND WALDA BESTHOFF SCULPTURE GARDEN

No matter where your eyes take you in the Sydney and Walda Besthoff Sculpture Garden at City Park, beauty abounds.

An extension of the New Orleans Museum of Art, the 5-acre garden comprises more than 60 sculptures situated among winding footpaths, reflecting lagoons, ancient live oaks, and pedestrian bridges. Among them are Robert Indiana's *Love, Red Blue*; Henry Moore's *Reclining Mother and Child*; Pierre-Auguste Renoir's *Venus Victorious*; and George Rodrigue's *Blue Dog*.

Other contemporary artists whose works are represented in the garden include Ida Kohlmeyer, Gaston Lachaise, Jean-Michel Othoniel, Yaacov Agam, and Joel Shapiro.

Open since 2003, the sculpture garden is named for New Orleans philanthropists and art collectors Sydney and Walda Besthoff, who through their private foundation donated most of the works that fill the garden. The foundation is dedicated to cultivating public interest in contemporary sculpture, and the garden—free and open to the public seven days a week—has served as a conduit to fulfilling that mission.

The museum offers a free audio tour accessible though visitors' cell phones. Additional programming includes yoga and Tai Chi classes, school field trips, a spring Easter-egg hunt, and the annual "Love in the Garden" fundraiser.

marked, so bring along this book and/or the official park map, available at **neworleanscitypark .com/in-the-park/city-park-map**.

● **Begin your walk at North Hennessey Street and City Park Avenue. Take note of the trees, especially the majestic, moss-dripping live oaks, which the park considers its pride and joy. The park boasts the oldest grove of mature live oaks in the world, and some—like the McDonogh and Anseman Oaks—are approximately 600–800 years old. Although City Park lost 2,000 of its 20,000 trees in Katrina, more than 5,000 new trees have been planted since. In addition to live oaks, you'll see bald cypress, magnolia, and other tree species. Feel free to wander through the maze of trees and take a closer look. You'll be glad you did.**

● Return to the walkway and, facing City Park Avenue, turn right, then walk one block to Anseman Avenue. Enter the park on Anseman through the Pizzati Gate, and cross the Anseman Bridge over Bayou Metairie, one of the many lagoons that wind through the park. The bridge, built in 1938 to replace the original 1928 structure, is named in honor of Victor Anseman, who, as the park's first executive committee chairman and volunteer manager, earned the title "Father of City Park."

● At Dreyfous Avenue, turn right and continue walking past two of the park's most historic landmarks—the Peristyle and the Popp Bandstand. The Peristyle, a Neoclassical open-air pavilion with a colonnade, was built in 1907 as a party place. It has undergone numerous renovations over the years, and today it is one of the park's most popular wedding and photo-taking venues. The Classical Greek–style Popp Bandstand went up in 1917. Designed by noted New Orleans architect Emile Weil, it features 12 granite columns topped with a bronze dome. In its infancy, it served as an outdoor theater for some of the earliest moving pictures, and dozens of musicians, including John Philip Sousa, have performed here over the years. Between the Peristyle and Popp Bandstand is the Stanley Ray Playground, which features swings, slides, and climbing contraptions.

Across from the Peristyle is the Goldring-Woldenberg Great Lawn, a 3-acre green space that opened in 2010 as part of the park's master plan. Adorned with palms, brick pathways, swings, pavilions, and a fountain, the lawn is frequently the site of concerts such as the Louisiana Philharmonic Orchestra's annual Swing in the Oaks.

● Continue down Dreyfous past the Casino Building, a Spanish Mission–style structure built in 1913. Today, it's home to Morning Call, a 24-hour café known for its café au lait and sugar-laden beignets but which also serves Louisiana dishes such as jambalaya and red beans and rice.

● Continue on Dreyfous, cross the bridge, and turn left onto Dueling Oaks Drive. This will take you to Collins Diboll Circle, adjacent to the New Orleans Museum of Art. At the circle, turn right; then make another right onto Lelong Avenue, walk to the end of the block, and cross Lelong in front of the park's Wisner Boulevard entrance. Walk back toward the museum on the other side of Lelong. To your right is Big Lake, which opened in 2009, providing park-goers with yet another opportunity for recreation. The lake is surrounded by 25 acres of wildlife and wetlands and paths for jogging, walking, and biking. Both boats and bikes are available to rent.

● Consider a stop at the New Orleans Museum of Art, which boasts a permanent collection of nearly 40,000 objects. The museum is especially known for its French and American art, along with photography, glass, and African and Japanese works. It is also a popular venue for films, plays, lectures, children's art workshops, wellness activities, and live-music performances.

● Circle right around the museum, past Big Lake and onto Roosevelt Mall Street. (Be sure to follow a map, because some streets aren't marked.) Cross bridge and turn left on Victory Avenue. To your left is the 5-acre Sydney and Walda Besthoff Sculpture Garden, considered one of the most important sculpture installations in the United States (see sidebar). The garden is part of the New Orleans Museum of Art but does not charge admission.

● From the sculpture garden, continue down Victory past the New Orleans Botanical Garden. What began as the City Park Rose Garden in 1936 is today home to 2,000 varieties of plants from around the world, among them aquatics, roses, native plants, ornamental trees, shrubs, and perennials. Highlights include the New Orleans Historic Train Garden, the Yakumo Nihon Teien Japanese Garden, the Conservatory of the Two Sisters, the Pavilion of the Two Sisters, the Garden Study Center, the Lath House, and the Robert B. Haspel Stage. The Botanical Garden presents a variety of programming throughout the year, including garden shows, lectures, and concerts, such as "Thursdays at Twilight," a garden concert series that showcases some of the city's top musicians and bands.

● Next to the Botanical Garden is the park's iconic Storyland, a must-see playground filled with fairy-tale sculptures such as Humpty Dumpty, the Three Little Pigs, and the Cheshire Cat. Kids are invited to climb aboard Captain Hook's pirate ship, follow Pinocchio into the mouth of a whale, and race up Jack and Jill's Hill.

Adjacent to Storyland is Carousel Gardens, an amusement park with 16 rides, including an antique wooden carousel that dates back to 1906. The carousel has 56 animals (mostly flying horses) and two chariots. Listed on the National Register of Historic Places, it is one of only 100 hand-carved carousels in the United States and the only one in Louisiana. Other rides include bumper cars, a Tilt-A-Whirl, a Ferris wheel, the Musik Express, and a miniature train. Kiddie rides are available for the toddler set.

Across from Carousel Gardens is another post-Katrina addition: City Putt, a 36-hole miniature-golf complex with two courses. The Louisiana Course focuses on themes and cities from around the state; the New Orleans Course showcases streets and local icons such as Louis Armstrong and Mr. Bingle, a storied Christmas character (a snowman with an ice-cream-cone hat) associated with the old Maison Blanche department store.

● Continue down Victory two blocks to Stadium Drive and turn left. Walk another block back to Dreyfous and turn left. Take Dreyfous to Anseman, turn right, and exit the park. Turn left and return to the starting point.

Though not part of the park, Ralph's On the Park, directly across the street from the Anseman entrance, is yet another of the city's classy eateries. It's an upscale restaurant, so if you're not quite dressed for it, do consider it another time.

POINTS OF INTEREST

City Park neworleanscitypark.com, 1 Palm Drive, 504-482-4888

Morning Call neworleanscitypark.com/in-the-park/morning-call, 56 Dreyfous Drive, 504-300-1157

New Orleans Museum of Art noma.org, 1 Collins Diboll Circle, 504-658-4100

Sydney and Walda Besthoff Sculpture Garden noma.org, 1 Collins Diboll Circle, 504-658-4100

New Orleans Botanical Garden neworleanscitypark.com/botanical-garden, 3 Victory Ave., 504-483-4888

Storyland neworleanscitypark.com/in-the-park/storyland, 7 Victory Ave., 504-483-4888

Carousel Gardens Amusement Park neworleanscitypark.com/in-the-park/carousel-gardens, Victory Avenue, 504-483-9402

City Putt neworleanscitypark.com/in-the-park/city-putt, 8 Victory Ave., 504-483-9385

Ralph's On the Park ralphsonthepark.com, 900 City Park Ave., 504-488-1000

route summary

1. Begin walk at North Hennessey Street and City Park Avenue.
2. Facing City Park Avenue, turn right and walk one block to Anseman Avenue.
3. Turn right on Anseman and walk one block to Dreyfous Avenue.
4. Turn right and take Dreyfous to Dueling Oaks Drive.
5. Turn left, then right onto Collins Diboll Circle.
6. Circle right to Lelong Avenue.
7. Walk down Lelong to just before the Wisner Boulevard entrance.
8. Cross Lelong and walk back on the opposite side.
9. At the museum, circle right on Collins Diboll Circle.
10. Walk to rear of museum and cross Roosevelt Mall Street bridge.
11. Make a quick left on Victory Avenue.
12. Walk four blocks down Victory to Stadium Drive and turn left.
13. Walk one block to Dreyfous and turn left.
14. Walk two blocks to Anseman and turn right.
15. Walk one block and exit park.
16. Turn left at City Park Avenue and return to starting point.

Humpty Dumpty and Little Bo Peep greet guests at City Park's Storyland.

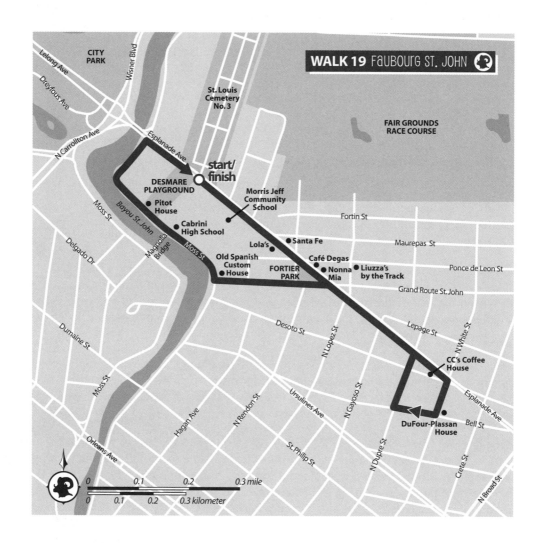

CITY PARK

Lelong Ave

Dreyfous Ave

N Carrollton Ave

Wisner Blvd

Esplanade Ave

St. Louis Cemetery No. 3

WALK 19 Faubourg St. John

FAIR GROUNDS RACE COURSE

start/ finish

DESMARE PLAYGROUND

● **Pitot House**

Moss St

Bayou St. John

Magnolia Bridge

Moss St

● **Cabrini High School**

Morris Jeff Community School

Fortin St

● **Lola's**

● **Santa Fe**

Maurepas St

Old Spanish Custom House ●

● **Café Degas**

FORTIER PARK

● **Nonna Mia**

● **Liuzza's by the Track**

Ponce de Leon St

Grand Route St. John

Delgado Dr

Desoto St

N Lopez St

Lepage St

N White St

Dumaine St

Moss St

Hagan Ave

N Rendon St

Ursulines Ave

N Gayoso St

CC's Coffee House ●

Esplanade Ave

Bell St

Orleans Ave

St Philip St

N Dupre St

DuFour-Plassan House

Crete St

N Broad St

0   0.1   0.2   0.3 mile
0   0.1   0.2   0.3 kilometer

19 FauBOUrG ST. JOHN: Beauty ON THE BaYOU

BOUNDARIES: Esplanade Ave., N. White St., Grand Route St. John, Moss St.
DISTANCE: 1.66 miles
PARKING: Free street parking
PUBLIC TRANSIT: Canal Streetcar (City Park/Museum Line)

Faubourg St. John, a section of the Esplanade Ridge Historic District, is one of those neighborhoods that, once you call it home, will likely be home forever. This community has it all, from stunning Creole cottages and Victorian mansions to parks, restaurants, cafés, and museums.

It is also a tight-knit community that, through the Faubourg St. John Neighborhood Association, has participated in numerous beautification projects, among them playground and park improvements, tree plantings, and neutral-ground maintenance.

Faubourg St. John dates back to 1708—10 years before the city of New Orleans was founded—when the French entered the city via Bayou St. John, which is connected to Lake Pontchartrain by way of the Gulf of Mexico and the Mississippi River. It eventually became the neighborhood of choice for the area's upper-class Creoles, particularly on Esplanade Avenue, an oak- and sycamore-lined street that stretches 2.5 miles from the river to City Park.

Just steps away from Bayou St. John and City Park, Faubourg St. John is within walking distance of such festivals as Bayou Boogaloo, held annually along Bayou St. John, and the New Orleans Jazz & Heritage Festival, held every year on the last weekend in April and the first weekend in May at the nearby Fair Grounds Race Course.

● **Begin at St. Louis Cemetery No. 3, established in 1854, when a yellow fever outbreak drove the need for more burial space. The cemetery is home to a number of "society tombs" owned by fraternal organizations, including those of the Dante Lodge of Masons, the Young Men's Benevolent Association, and the United Slavonian Benevolent Association. Before it was a cemetery, the site was a leper colony known as "Leper's Land."**

Across the street is Desmare Playground, one of the city's many neighborhood parks and playgrounds. Desmare has undergone numerous facelifts over the years, many of them courtesy of members of the Faubourg St. John Neighborhood Association, which holds annual fundraisers to help its cause. One of the biggest is the Porch Crawl, whereby homes and their porches are paired with area restaurants, and patrons stroll to each one, enjoying great food, drinks, and music.

● Walk one block to Cabrini High School, a Catholic girls' school named for St. Frances Xavier Cabrini, the first woman to establish a missionary order of women and the first American citizen to be canonized as a saint of the Catholic Church. The school opened in 1959 in what was then the Sacred Heart Orphan Asylum. Mother Cabrini raised the money for both the orphanage and the school, once saying, "The greatest heritage to a girl is a good education."

Next to Cabrini is the back of Our Lady of the Rosary Catholic Church, founded in 1907. The church, which faces Bayou St. John, had its majestic copper dome replated after Hurricane Katrina, and the dome is illuminated at night.

Morris Jeff Community School, at 3368 Esplanade, is one of dozens of charter schools that opened in New Orleans after Katrina. Morris Jeff is an International Baccalaureate school, offering a curriculum that focuses on creating a globally minded child. The school offers traditional academics with a focus on Spanish language, the arts, and community service. The Esplanade building is Morris Jeff's temporary home while construction takes place on the school's permanent facility on nearby South Lopez Street.

● The next stretch of blocks features two family-owned grocery stores, Terranova's Superette and Canseco's, along with restaurants such as Santa Fe, a Southwestern restaurant offering live jazz on Thursday and Sunday nights; Lola's, known for its paella and other Spanish fare; Café Degas, a French eatery with one of the best patio dining rooms in town; and Nonna Mia, a pizzeria that also serves classic Sicilian pasta dishes. Craving a po'boy? Head down Ponce de Leon Street to Liuzza's by the Track. On Ponce de Leon, you'll also find Fair Grinds, a coffeehouse; Lux, a day spa; and Swirl, a wine bar and market.

- From Café Degas, walk four blocks to 2821 Esplanade, a neo-Tudor style residence built in the 1920s. Next door, at 2809 Esplanade, is a Queen Anne–style home built in 1902. Known as the Cresson House, it is a favorite photo-taking spot.

- Cross Esplanade at North White Street in front of McDonogh City Park Academy, another of the city's many charter schools. On the opposite side of Esplanade, you'll pass CC's Coffee House, a great place to grab a latte or cappuccino. Continue on North White one block to the corner of Bell Street. The DuFour-Plassan House, at 1206 N. White, was built in 1870 and boasts one of the few wrought-iron cornstalk fences in New Orleans.

- Turn right on Bell and walk one block to North Dupre Street. Turn right on North Dupre, walk two blocks to Esplanade, and turn left. Walk three blocks to Grand Route St. John. As you walk down Esplanade, you'll notice an array of architectural styles from classic bungalows to Greek Revivals, many adorned with black-and-gold Jazz Fest flags. Because the neighborhood is built on naturally high ground, it escaped the flooding that ravaged so many other New Orleans neighborhoods in Hurricane Katrina.

- Turn left onto Grand Route St. John in front of Fortier Park, an intimate green space that boasts sculptures, palms, and other lush greenery. The park is named for Alcee Fortier, a philanthropist and professor of romance languages at Tulane University.

- Walk four blocks to Moss Street on Grand Route St. John, one of the neighborhood's most beautifully maintained streets. Turn right at Moss in front of the meandering Bayou St. John. This is believed to be the approximate spot where, back in the 18th and early 19th centuries, travelers disembarked from boats as they made their way into the city via Grand Route St. John. At the corner of Moss and Grand Route St. John is the Old Spanish Custom House, which was built in 1784 and is the oldest building in the neighborhood.

- Continue walking down Moss past Bayou St. John Bed and Breakfast, a 150-year-old house-turned-inn at 1318 Moss. Another historic structure is the Holy Rosary rectory (1342 Moss), a Greek Revival mansion built in 1834.

● As you continue walking, take note of the pedestrian-only bridge that crosses the bayou in front of Cabrini High School. Known as the Magnolia Bridge, it's a popular spot for parties and fishing. Next to Cabrini High, at 1440 Moss, is the Pitot House, an 18th-century Creole Colonial plantation that serves as the home of the Louisiana Landmarks Society. The organization works to promote historic preservation through education and advocacy and invites the public to tour the house and learn about life along the bayou since the earliest days of the settlement. Each year, the society hosts a series of fundraisers called Vino on the Bayou, featuring wine tastings, music, and food.

● From Pitot House, continue down Moss and circle right as you head back to Esplanade. Across the bayou are City Park and the New Orleans Museum of Art (see the previous walk). Note the equestrian statue of Confederate general P. G. T. Beauregard at the entrance of the park. Cross Esplanade, turn right, and return to the starting point at St. Louis Cemetery No. 3.

POINTS OF INTEREST

St. Louis Cemetery No. 3 saveourcemeteries.org, 3421 Esplanade Ave., 504-482-5065

Desmare Playground 3456 Esplanade Ave. between Esplanade and Moss Street

Cabrini High School cabrinihigh.com, 1400 Moss St., 504-482-1193

Our Lady of the Rosary Catholic Church ourladyoftherosary-no.com, 3368 Esplanade Ave., 504-488-2659

Lola's lolasneworleanscom, 3312 Esplanade Ave., 504-488-6946

Santa Fe santafenola.com, 3201 Esplanade Ave., 504-948-0077

Liuzza's by the Track liuzzasnola.com, 1518 N. Lopez St., 504-218-7888

Café Degas cafedegas.com, 3127 Esplanade Ave., 504-945-5635

Nonna Mia nonnamia.net, 3125 Esplanade Ave., 504-948-1717

CC's Coffee House ccscoffee.com, 2800 Esplanade Ave., 504-482-9865

Fortier Park Bounded by Esplanade Avenue, Grand Route St. John, and Mystery Street

Pitot House louisianalandmarks.org, 1440 Moss St., 504-482-0312

rouTE SUMMArY

1. Begin walk on Esplanade Avenue in front of St. Louis No. 3 Cemetery.
2. Walk 10 blocks to North White Street and cross Esplanade.
3. Walk one block to Bell Street and turn right.
4. Walk one block to North Dupre Street and turn right.
5. Walk two blocks to Esplanade and turn left.
6. Walk three blocks to Grand Route St. John.
7. Turn left and walk four blocks to Moss Street.
8. Turn right and continue on Moss.
9. Circle right on Moss and walk to Esplanade.
10. Cross Esplanade and turn right.
11. Return to starting point in front of cemetery.

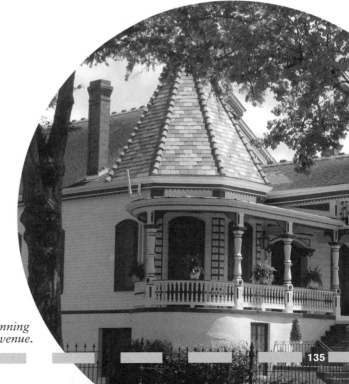

The Cresson House is just one of many stunning homes that line Esplanade Avenue.

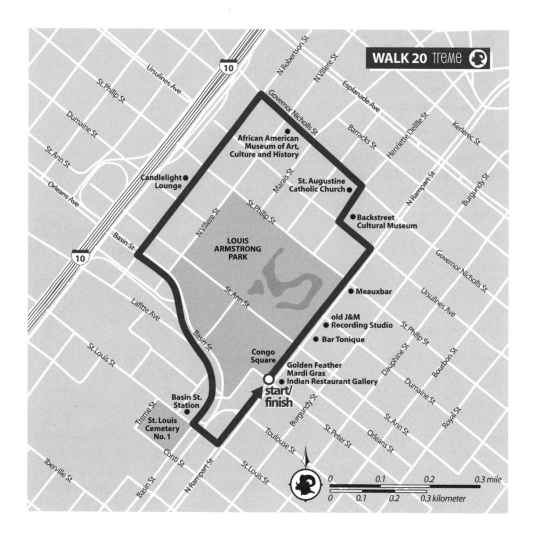

Ursulines Ave

St. Philip St

Dumaine St

St. Ann St

Orleans Ave

N Robertson St

N Villere St

Esplanade Ave

Governor Nicholls St

Barracks St

Henriette Delille St

Kerlerec St

Burgundy St

N Rampart St

African American
Museum of Art,
Culture and History

Candlelight
Lounge

Marais St

St. Philip St

St. Augustine
Catholic Church

Backstreet
Cultural Museum

Governor Nicholls St

N Villere St

Basin St

LOUIS
ARMSTRONG
PARK

Ursulines Ave

St. Philip St

Meauxbar

old J&M
Recording Studio

Bar Tonique

Dauphine St

Bourbon St

Royal St

St. Ann St

Lafitte Ave

Basin St

St. Ann St

St. Louis St

Congo
Square

Golden Feather
Mardi Gras
Indian Restaurant Gallery

start/
finish

Dumaine St

St. Ann St

Basin St.
Station

Treme St

St. Louis
Cemetery
No. 1

Burgundy St

St. Peter St

Orleans St

Iberville St

Conti St

N Rampart St

St. Louis St

Toulouse St

0   0.1   0.2   0.3 mile

0   0.1   0.2   0.3 kilometer

20 Treme: More Than an HBO Series

BOUNDARIES: **Basin St., N. Rampart St., Governor Nicholls St., N. Robertson St.**
DISTANCE: **1.46 miles**
PARKING: **Metered parking on N. Rampart St.**
PUBLIC TRANSIT: **RTA Buses #57 (Franklin), #88 (St. Claude/Jackson Barracks), and #91 (Jackson-Esplanade)**

For countless Mardi Gras revelers, celebrating Fat Tuesday means packing up the family, picking up some Popeye's, and heading to St. Charles Avenue to enjoy a day of parades. For others, it means heading out of town and not returning until the last strand of beads has been tossed.

Then there are those who wouldn't spend the day anywhere else but in Treme, (prounouced treh-MAY), the oldest African American neighborhood in the United States and the cultural heart of New Orleans. In Treme, Mardi Gras means second-line parades, exquisitely costumed Mardi Gras Indians, and the North Side Skull and Bones Gang, which has been waking up the neighborhood on Fat Tuesday since 1819.

Unless you're in New Orleans for Mardi Gras, you won't have the chance to experience that exuberating scene. But on any given day in Treme, you might witness a jazz funeral, a spontaneous second-line parade, or a wandering musician blowing his horn just because.

Such scenes played out weekly on the critically acclaimed HBO series *Treme*, which chronicled the struggles of musicians and other residents in the months and years following Katrina. The series lasted only three seasons (2010–2013), but it exposed to the world one of America's most fascinating neighborhoods.

● **Begin at Congo Square in Louis Armstrong Park.** The 31-acre park includes the New Orleans Municipal Auditorium, the Mahalia Jackson Theater for the Performing Arts, and Congo Square, where in the 18th century slaves would gather on Sundays—their day off—to set up market and play music. In addition to walking paths, lagoons, and gardens, the park contains a statue of Armstrong, a bust of jazz saxophonist Sidney Bechet, and a sculpture of Buddy Bolden, a cornetist often referred to as the Father of Jazz. As one might expect, the park is home to numerous music festivals, including

ST. AUGUSTINE CATHOLIC CHURCH

One of the oldest African American Catholic parishes in the United States, St. Augustine was established on the property of a one-time plantation as the result of a decision by Bishop Antoine Blanc to allow free people of color a place to worship.

One of the more fascinating stories about the church is the so-called War of the Pews. Just before the church was dedicated in 1842, people of color began buying pews for their family members. White people responded by buying their own pews, their goal to buy more than the "colored" members. Their campaign failed, for the free people of color ended up buying three pews to every one bought by the whites. In what the church described as an unprecedented social, political, and religious move, the free people of color also bought the pews of both side-aisles and gave them to the slaves as their exclusive place of worship, a first in the history of slavery in the United States. According to the church's website, the mix of the pews resulted in the most integrated congregation in the United States.

In 2004, St. Augustine dedicated the Tomb of the Unknown Slave, described on a bronze plaque as a "shrine consisting of grave crosses, chains and shackles to the memory of the nameless, faceless, turf-less Africans who met an untimely death in Faubourg Treme." The plaque goes on to say, "This St. Augustine/Treme shrine honors all slaves buried throughout the United States and those slaves in particular who lie beneath the ground of Treme in unmarked, unknown graves."

In 2008, the church was placed on the African American Heritage Trail for historic sites of cultural significance in Louisiana. You may arrange a tour by calling the church rectory at 504-525-5934. Mass, held every Sunday at 10 a.m., is yet another way to experience this historical landmark.

the Louisiana Cajun-Zydeco Festival and Jazz in the Park, a series of concerts featuring such greats as the Treme Brass Band, Irma Thomas, and Charmaine Neville.

Across the street, at 704 N. Rampart, is the Golden Feather Mardi Gras Indian Restaurant Gallery, where you can learn about Indian culture while enjoying such traditional fare as the Big Chief (fish smothered in onions, tomatoes, and African spices and served over brown or white rice), the Bamboula (veggie gumbo), and Hu Ta Nay (stuffed shrimp with crabmeat dressing). The restaurant, which has an art gallery and gift shop, often hosts lectures and sewing demonstrations by Mardi Gras Indian Chief Shaka Zulu.

- Down the block on North Rampart are two of this area's trendiest bars, Bar Tonique and Meauxbar. Bar Tonique boasts a menu of original, adapted, and classic cocktails, along with eclectic beer and wine selections. Meauxbar has equally impressive selection of libations along with appetizers and entrees such as goat cheese tart, French-onion grilled cheese, and hanger steak au poivre.

- At North Rampart and Dumaine, between Bar Tonique and Meauxbar, is the site of the old J&M Recording Studio, considered the birthplace of rhythm and blues. Among the greats who recorded there were local luminaries Fats Domino and Aaron Neville, as well as stars such as Little Richard, Jerry Lee Lewis, and Ray Charles.

- Walk to the end of the park, then another block to Ursulines Avenue, and turn left. Walk one block to Henriette Delille Street and turn right. This street is named for the founder of the Catholic order of the Sisters of the Holy Family in New Orleans. Delille, a free woman of color, devoted her life to serving the poor.

- In the middle of the block is the Backstreet Cultural Museum, which opened in 1999 to preserve and perpetuate the cultural traditions of New Orleans's African American community. The museum has the world's most comprehensive collection of artifacts related to the masking and parading traditions of the city's African American community. They include exhibits on Mardi Gras Indians, jazz funerals, social aid and pleasure clubs, Baby Dolls (female maskers in frilly attire), and Skull and Bone gangs, as well as filmed records of more than 500 events. In addition to hosting music and dance performances, conducting outreach programs, and creating an annual book that documents the year's jazz funerals, the museum serves as the starting and ending point for second-line parades and as an assembly spot for the North Side Skull and Bone Gang and Mardi Gras Indians on Fat Tuesday.

- Walk a half-block to Governor Nicholls Street and turn left. At the corner is St. Augustine's Catholic Church (1210 Governor Nicholls), the oldest African American Roman Catholic parish in the United States (see sidebar).

- Continue on Governor Nicholls for two and a half blocks. The New Orleans African American Museum of Art, Culture and History opened in 2000, its mission "to preserve, interpret and promote the African American cultural heritage of New Orleans, with a particular emphasis on the Treme community." The museum offers walking tours covering such landmarks as St. Augustine's Church, Congo Square, and a row of Creole cottages. As of this writing, the museum had closed for a $6 million renovation but was continuing the walking tours.

- Walk one and a half blocks to North Robertson Street, turn left, then walk two and a half blocks to the Candlelight Lounge, a legendary Treme music club. It's a dive, but a dive worth visiting, especially on Wednesday nights, when you can get free red beans and rice while enjoying the rollicking sounds of the Treme Brass Band. The band, led by snare drummer Benny Jones Sr., starts doing its thing around 9 p.m., and the place is almost always packed. Adjacent to the Candlelight is Tuba Fats Square, named for Anthony "Tuba Fats" Lacen, a founding member of the Dirty Dozen Brass Band and, until his death in 2004, the city's most famous tuba player. Every year, on the Tuesday night after the New Orleans Jazz & Heritage Festival, some of the city's top brass musicians converge on Tuba Fats Square for Tuba Fats Tuesday, a musical celebration in Lacen's memory.

- Walk two and a half blocks to Basin Street, cross Basin, and turn left. Circle right around Basin past the Basin St. Station, a restored Southern Railway station that now serves as a visitor-information and cultural center. If you have time, stop in and learn about New Orleans through exhibits, murals, art, music, crafts, and entertainment.

- Continue on Basin to St. Louis Street. At the corner is St. Louis Cemetery No. 1. Founded in 1789 and listed on the National Register of Historic Places, it is the oldest existing cemetery in New Orleans. It's also the final resting spot for voodoo queen Marie Laveau; Étienne de Boré, the first mayor of New Orleans, who also produced the first granulated sugar; and Paul Morphy, a world-renowned chess player. If you're interested in walking through the cemetery, we strongly advise taking a formal tour. One of the best is conducted by Save Our Cemeteries, a nonprofit group dedicated to preserving the city's historic burial grounds. Ninety percent of the ticket price goes to cemetery restoration, education, and advocacy.

- Cross Basin Street at St. Louis and walk one block to North Rampart Street. Turn left at North Rampart and continue back to the starting point at Louis Armstrong Park.

POINTS OF INTEREST

Louis Armstrong Park nola.gov/parks-and-parkways/parks-squares/congo-square-louis
-armstrong-park, 701 N. Rampart St., 504-658-3200

Golden Feather Mardi Gras Indian Restaurant Gallery goldenfeatherneworleans.com,
704 N. Rampart St., 504-266-2339

Bar Tonique bartonique.com, 820 N. Rampart St., 504-324-6045

Meauxbar meauxbar.com, 942 N. Rampart St., 504-569-9979

Backstreet Cultural Museum backstreetmuseum.org, 1116 Henriette Delille St.,
504-522-4806

St. Augustine Catholic Church staugustinecatholicchurch-neworleans.org,
1210 Governor Nicholls St., 504-525-5934

African American Museum of Art, Culture and History noaam.org,
1418 Governor Nicholls St., 504-566-1136

Candlelight Lounge 925 N. Robertson St., 504-525-4748

Basin St. Station basinststation.com, 501 Basin St.,
504-293-2600

St. Louis Cemetery No. 1 saveourcemeteries.org,
320 N. Claiborne Ave., 504-596-3050

ROUTE SUMMARY

1. Begin walk at Louis Armstrong Park.
2. Walk five blocks to Ursulines Avenue and turn left.
3. Walk one block to Henriette Delille Street and turn right.
4. Walk one block to Governor Nicholls Street and turn left.
5. Walk four blocks to North Robertson Street and turn left.
6. Walk five blocks to Basin Street and turn left.
7. Walk four blocks to St. Louis Street.
8. Cross Basin at St. Louis and walk one block to North Rampart Street.
9. Turn left on North Rampart; return to starting point.

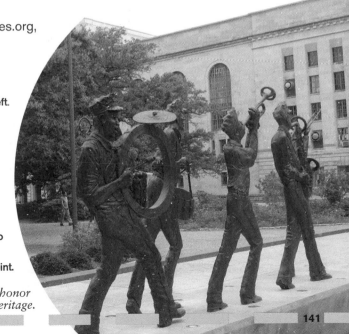

These sculptures in Armstrong Park honor the city's rich jazz heritage.

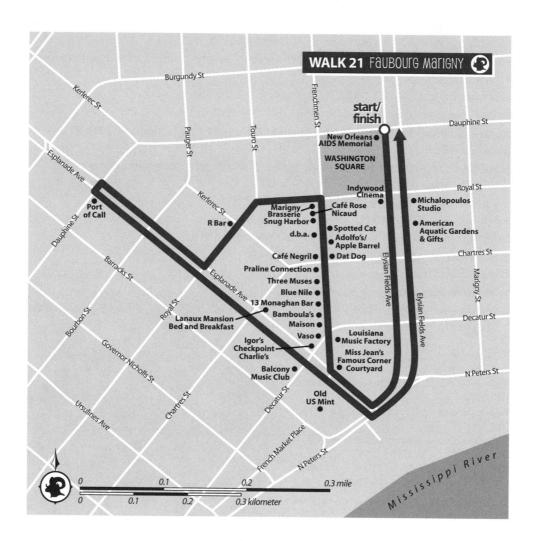

start/
finish

New Orleans
AIDS Memorial

WASHINGTON
SQUARE

Indywood
Cinema

Michalopoulos
Studio

Marigny
Brasserie
Snug Harbor

Café Rose
Nicaud

American
Aquatic Gardens
& Gifts

R Bar

Spotted Cat

d.b.a.

Adolfo's/
Apple Barrel

Café Negril

Dat Dog

Praline Connection

Three Muses

Blue Nile

13 Monaghan Bar

Bamboula's

Lanaux Mansion
Bed and Breakfast

Maison

Vaso

Igor's
Checkpoint
Charlie's

Louisiana
Music Factory

Miss Jean's
Famous Corner
Courtyard

Balcony
Music Club

Old
US Mint

Burgundy St

Kerlerec St

Esplanade Ave

Port
of Call

Dauphine St

Barracks St

Bourbon St

Royal St

Governor Nicholls St

Chartres St

Ursulines Ave

Pauger St

Touro St

Frenchmen St

Kerlerec St

Esplanade Ave

Royal St

Decatur St

French Market Place

N Peters St

Dauphine St

Royal St

Chartres St

Decatur St

N Peters St

Elysian Fields Ave

Elysian Fields Ave

Marigny St

Mississippi River

0		0.1		0.2		0.3 mile

0	0.1	0.2	0.3 kilometer

21 Faubourg Marigny: Music Lover's Delight

BOUNDARIES: Elysian Fields Ave., Esplanade Ave., Dauphine St., N. Peters St.
DISTANCE: 1.54 miles
PARKING: Metered parking, parking lots, some free street parking
PUBLIC TRANSIT: Riverfront Streetcar

Ask local music lovers where they enjoy listening to jazz, blues, rock, and funk, and you're sure to hear names like Tipitina's in Uptown, Howlin' Wolf in the Warehouse District, and the Rock 'N' Bowl in Carrollton. You may also hear names like Snug Harbor, Blue Nile, and Spotted Cat, three of a bounty of clubs that make up the fun and funky music scene on Frenchmen Street in historic Faubourg Marigny.

The people you ask may or may not share those details, however: Locals tend to want to keep the Marigny—as it's commonly called—to themselves, though even they recognize that it's becoming a hot spot for tourists, particularly those looking for fun off the beaten path.

Just downriver of the French Quarter, the Marigny (MARE-uh-nee) is one of the coolest, most eclectic neighborhoods in all of New Orleans, and that's saying a lot, considering the uniqueness of each one. On Frenchmen Street, the main drag, you'll find tattoo parlors, art galleries, restaurants, a coffeehouse, a bike shop, a used-book store, and, the biggest draw of all, music clubs. It's a popular "Hollywood South" locale as well, with the TV crime drama *NCIS: New Orleans* and the 2014 flick *Chef* among recent productions shooting here.

But Faubourg Marigny is far more than an entertainment district. It has an equally fascinating history, its development going back to 1805 when millionaire developer Bernard de Marigny (who popularized the game of craps) subdivided his family's plantation to create what is considered New Orleans's first suburb. Although the neighborhood began to deteriorate in the 1950s, renewed interest in its history, culture, and architecture led to its rebirth in the early 1970s, when it was placed on the National Register of Historic Places. Today, the Marigny is thriving, with beautifully restored Victorian shotguns and Creole cottages, many painted in eye-popping colors, lining the streets.

● **Begin at Elysian Fields Avenue and Dauphine Street, in front of Washington Square, a 2.5-acre park that serves as a popular hangout for residents and venue for festivals,**

THE OLD US MINT

In a neighborhood brimming with music clubs, there might not be a better place to learn about the history of jazz—and listen to it—than the Old US Mint, one of 12 sites that make up the Louisiana State Museum.

Once used to mint both Union and Confederate currency, the Greek Revival–style structure became a museum in 1981, boasting such permanent exhibits as "New Orleans Jazz," which features instruments, sheet music, and memorabilia depicting the history of the genre in New Orleans, along with a photography gallery showcasing some of the city's premiere musicians.

Music at the Mint is a series of jazz concerts that take place throughout the year and during some of the area's biggest events—including the French Quarter Festival and Satchmo SummerFest, an annual tribute to Louisiana's own Louis Armstrong. Performers have included the Barbarin Family of Jazz, singer-songwriter Alexandra Scott, and rock band Rejected Youth Nation, part of the next generation of New Orleans music.

In addition to the jazz exhibits, the Old US Mint features an exhibit on the Mississippi River and another on the internationally acclaimed Arts and Crafts pottery produced by students at Sophie Newcomb College of Tulane University from 1895 to 1940. In addition, the museum houses the Louisiana Historical Center, the New Orleans Jazz Club Collections, and the New Orleans Mint Performing Arts Center.

art markets, and other events. One of the highlights of the square is the New Orleans AIDS Memorial, a series of glass discs depicting the faces of AIDS in the city.

● Walk four blocks to North Peters Street. In the first block, just past Royal Street, is the neighborhood's newest addition: the Indywood Cinema, a sort of hole-in-the-wall independent movie theater housed in an old laundromat. The theater specializes in Louisiana-made films and can be rented out for parties. In the fall of 2014, part-time New Orleans resident Solange Knowles—sister of Beyoncé—held one of her pre-wedding parties here. Also in this block is I. J. Reilly and Sons Knick-Knacks and Curi-osities, which sells such items as jewelry made out of recycled materials. The shop's address is 632 Elysian Fields—the same address where Stella and Stanley Kowalski lived in *A Streetcar Named Desire*—and it's named after Ignatius J. Reilly, the rotund protagonist of *A Confederacy of Dunces.*

● Circle right to Esplanade Avenue in front of Hotel de la Monnaie. Walk another block and veer right on Frenchmen, in front of Miss Jean's Famous Corner Courtyard, the first of several music clubs that you'll pass over the next three blocks. At the end of the block on the right is the Louisiana Music Factory, a music store that occasionally hosts free concerts. To the left across Frenchmen is Vaso, a so-called ultralounge with brass bands, DJs, and food.

● Continue on the second block of Frenchmen past The Maison, a live-music venue and restaurant; Bamboula's, which combines the blues with Caribbean cuisine; 13 Monaghan Bar & Restaurant, where the specialty menu item is Tater Tot nachos ("Tachos"); and Blue Nile, which stages funk, blues, soul, and brass-band shows in a building dating back to 1832. Three Muses is a restaurant and music club where you can munch on such fare as duck-pastrami pizza or curried chickpea–crusted scallops while taking in the sounds of singer and trombonist Glen David Andrews or pianist Tom McDermott.

At the corner of Frenchmen and Chartres Streets is The Praline Connection, which before opening in 1990 ran a home-delivery service targeting working women who were too busy to cook for their families. The soul food eatery at 542 Frenchmen specializes in Southern cuisine, from fried chicken to red beans and rice. Of course, pralines (pro-nounced PRAW-leenz as opposed to PRAY-leenz) are its specialty. Inside the restaurant is a separate shop where you can buy pralines, seasonings, sauces, and other goodies.

● Cross Chartres Street and continue down Frenchmen past even more clubs and restaurants, including Café Negril, a reggae club known for its dancing atmosphere; Dat Dog, famous for its gourmet hot dogs and sausages; Café Rose Nicaud, a coffee-house named for the first known coffee vendor in New Orleans; Spotted Cat, known for its old-time swing jazz; and d.b.a., where regular performers include some of the hottest names in New Orleans music, among them Walter "Wolfman" Washington, Jon Cleary, the Soul Rebels, and the Treme Brass Band. At the legendary Snug Harbor, contemporary jazz greats Charmaine Neville, Donald Harrison, Ellis Marsalis, and the Uptown Jazz Orchestra pack in the crowds. And at the corner of Frenchmen and Royal, Marigny Brasserie serves up a menu of Creole cuisine along with such entertainers as the Pfister Sisters, Paul Sanchez, and the Washboard Chaz Blues Trio.

Apple Barrel rounds out the medley of music clubs. Adolfo's, on the second floor of Apple Barrel, is a Creole-Italian eatery whose signature dish is corn-and-crab cannelloni. If you're visiting Frenchmen on Thursday through Sunday nights, stop by the Frenchmen Art Market, in the lot next to Spotted Cat.

- Turn left on Royal Street and walk one block to the intersection of Royal and Touro Street. Continue down Royal, cross Kerlerec Street, walk another block to Esplanade Avenue, and turn right. This is a mostly residential area, but a number of bed-and-breakfasts and guest houses line this stretch. Among them is the Royal Inn (1431 Royal), home of the hopping R Bar, a dive that draws huge crowds for its affordable drinks and funky vibe.

- Cross Esplanade at Dauphine Street, turn left, and begin walking back down Esplanade to the starting point. Don't be surprised to see a crowd of people standing in front of 838 Esplanade. This is Port of Call, which, even with the proliferation of burger restaurants around town, is still considered one of the city's best.

- You'll pass several Victorian mansions on both sides of Esplanade, including the Lanaux Mansion (to your left at 547 Esplanade), an 1879 Renaissance Revival home that *Forbes* magazine has called one of the best bed-and-breakfasts in the country. The exterior of the inn and its lobby were featured in the Brad Pitt film *The Curious Case of Benjamin Button.* The inn's decor includes original furniture and wallpapers from 1879, as well as Civil War memorabilia. Registered guests can arrange for a tour upon their arrival.

  Music venues abound on this stretch as well, among them Igor's Checkpoint Charlie's (501 Esplanade Ave.), which specializes in alternative-rock and metal bands, and the Balcony Music Club (BMC), at the corner of Esplanade and Decatur Street, which features blues, funk, and R&B bands.

- From BMC, cross Decatur and you'll be in front of the Old US Mint, home of the Music at the Mint jazz series and one of several museums that make up the Louisiana State Museum system (see sidebar). Built in 1835, the Greek Revival building served as a mint for both the Union and the Confederacy. Today, it's home to exhibits on New Orleans jazz, Newcomb pottery, and the Mississippi River.

- Cross Esplanade at North Peters Street, then circle left on North Peters, which becomes Elysian Fields Avenue heading north. Cross on Elysian Fields where North Peters picks up again heading right, but be cautious, as this is an especially busy intersection.

- Bear left on Elysian Fields and walk four blocks north to Dauphine. During this stretch you'll pass American Aquatic Gardens & Gifts, which sells rare water lilies and other plants, and Michalopoulos Studio, the home of celebrated New Orleans artist James Michalopoulos (open to the public Thursday–Sunday, 11 a.m.–4 p.m).

- Cross on Elysian Fields at Dauphine and return to the starting point at Washington Square.

POINTS OF INTEREST

Washington Square nola.gov/parks-and-parkways/parks-squares /washington-square, Bounded by Elysian Fields Avenue and Frenchmen, Dauphine, and Royal Streets; 504-658-3200

Indywood Cinema indywood.org, 628 Elysian Fields Ave., 504-345-8804

I. J. Reilly's Knick-Knacks and Curiosities ijreillys.squarespace.com, 632 Elysian Fields Ave., 504-304-7928

Miss Jean's Famous Corner Courtyard tinyurl.com/missjeans, 437 Esplanade Ave., 504-252-4800

Louisiana Music Factory louisianamusic factory.com, 421 Frenchmen St., 504-586-1094

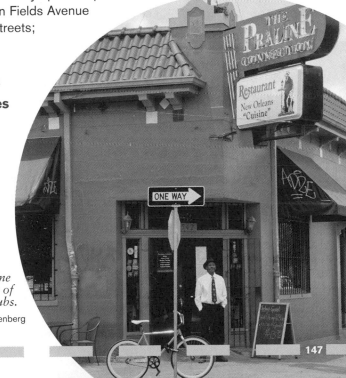

Enjoy the Southern cuisine at The Praline Connection, then dance off the calories at one of the area's many music clubs.

Photo: Donna Goldenberg

147

Vaso facebook.com/vasonola, 500 Frenchmen St., 504-272-0929

The Maison maisonfrenchmen.com, 508 Frenchmen St., 504-371-5543

Bamboula's bamboulasnola.com, 514 Frenchmen St., 504-944-8461

13 Monaghan Bar 13monaghan.com, 517 Frenchmen St., 504-942-1345

Blue Nile bluenilelive.com, 532 Frenchmen St., 504-948-2583

Three Muses 3musesnola.com, 536 Frenchmen St., 504-252-4801

The Praline Connection pralineconnection.com, 542 Frenchmen St., 504-943-3934

Dat Dog datdognola.com, 601 Frenchmen St., 504-309-3362

Café Negril 606 Frenchmen St., 504-944-4744

Apple Barrel tinyurl.com/applebarrelnola, 609 Frenchmen St., 504-949-9399

Adolfo's tinyurl.com/adolfosnola, 611 Frenchmen St., 504-948-3800

d.b.a. dbaneworleans.com, 618 Frenchmen St., 504-942-3731

Spotted Cat spottedcatmusicclub.com, 623 Frenchmen St. (no phone)

Snug Harbor snugjazz.com, 626 Frenchmen St., 504-949-0696

Café Rose Nicaud caferosenicaud.com, 632 Frenchmen St., 504-949-3300

Marigny Brasserie marignybrasserie.com, 640 Frenchmen St., 504-945-4472

R Bar royalstreetinn.com/r-bar, 1431 Royal St., 504-948-7499

Port of Call portofcallnola.com, 838 Esplanade Ave., 504-523-0120

Lanaux Mansion Bed and Breakfast lanauxmansion.com, 547 Esplanade Ave., 504-330-2826

Igor's Checkpoint Charlie's 501 Esplanade Ave., 504-281-4847

Balcony Music Club 1331 Decatur St., 504-522-2940

Old US Mint crt.state.la.us/museum/properties/usmint, 400 Esplanade Ave., 504-568-6993

American Aquatic Gardens americanaquaticgardens.com, 621 Elysian Fields Ave., 504-944-0410

Michalopoulos Studio michalopoulos.com, 527 Elysian Fields Ave., 504-558-0505

route summary

1. Begin at Elysian Fields Avenue and Dauphine Street.
2. Walk four blocks to North Peters Street.
3. Circle right onto Esplanade Avenue.
4. Walk one block to Frenchmen Street and turn right.
5. Walk three blocks to Royal Street and turn left.
6. Walk two blocks to Esplanade and turn right.
7. Walk two blocks to Dauphine Street and cross Esplanade.
8. Turn left on Esplanade.
9. Walk five blocks to North Peters and turn left.
10. Walk one block to Elysian Fields.
11. Cross North Peters on Elysian Fields and bear left.
12. Walk four blocks to Dauphine.
13. Cross Dauphine on Elysian Fields and return to starting point.

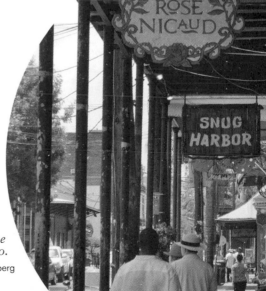

Snug Harbor is one of the oldest jazz clubs in the Marigny. You can get a great burger there, too.
Photo: Donna Goldenberg

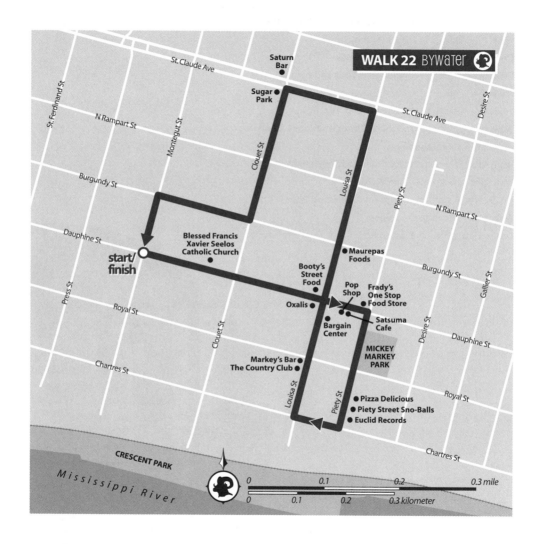

WALK 22 BYWATER

Saturn Bar

St. Claude Ave

St. Ferdinand St

N Rampart St

Montegut St

Clouet St

Sugar Park

Burgundy St

Louisa St

St. Claude Ave

Desire St

Piety St

N Rampart St

Dauphine St

Blessed Francis Xavier Seelos Catholic Church

start/ finish

Press St

Maurepas Foods

Burgundy St

Gallier St

Booty's Street Food

Pop Shop

Frady's One Stop Food Store

Royal St

Oxalis

Clouet St

Bargain Center

Satsuma Cafe

Desire St

Dauphine St

MICKEY MARKEY PARK

Chartres St

Markey's Bar The Country Club

Louisa St

Piety St

Pizza Delicious

Piety Street Sno-Balls

Euclid Records

Royal St

Chartres St

CRESCENT PARK

Mississippi River

0   0.1   0.2   0.3 mile

0   0.1   0.2   0.3 kilometer

22 BYWATER: HIPSTERS' HAVEN

BOUNDARIES: St. Claude Ave., Chartres St., Piety St., Montegut St.
DISTANCE: 1.29 miles
PARKING: Free street parking
PUBLIC TRANSIT: RTA Bus #5 (Marigny-Bywater)

A lot of words have been tossed about to describe the Bywater section of New Orleans, and, well, most of them are true. The neighborhood along the Mississippi River between Faubourg Marigny and the Industrial Canal is perhaps the funkiest, edgiest, most bohemian 'hood in New Orleans. And yeah, we may as well throw in the term *hipster*, too.

The evolution of Bywater as the city's "it" neighborhood began after Hurricane Katrina in 2005, and it has been exploding in popularity ever since. Because of its higher elevation along the river, it escaped the flooding that destroyed so many other parts of town. As a result, the so-called "Sliver by the River" became a magnet for folks looking for new places to lay roots. Of late, Bywater has become a haven for newcomers, along with artists and musicians.

The houses alone make this neighborhood something special. We're not talking mansions— we're talking Creole cottages and shotgun doubles painted in eye-popping shades of purple, orange, and blue, and trimmed in equally vibrant colors. The houses are so much fun to look at that one could easily miss everything else this neighborhood has to offer, from restaurants and music clubs to arts venues and parks. Bywater's newest addition, as of February 2014, is Crescent Park, a 1.4-mile linear park built along the river.

● **Start your walk at the corner of Montegut and Dauphine Streets. Walk to 3053 Dauphine, home of the Blessed Francis Xavier Seelos Catholic Church. Listed on the National Register of Historic Places, the church opened in 1838 as St. Vincent de Paul Parish but was renamed in 2001 for Seelos, a Redemptorist priest known for his devotion to the poor and abandoned. Two years later, the interior of the church was destroyed by a fire but has since been restored. The church has stunning stained-glass windows and a massive pipe organ donated by a group of Seattle-based churches whose volunteers had come to New Orleans to help in the Katrina recovery.**

CRESCENT PARK

It was eight years in the making, but when Crescent Park opened in February 2014 along the Mississippi River, it was hailed as a major step in the city's revitalization. City officials said it also fulfilled their mission of returning the riverfront to the people.

Stretching from Bywater to the Marigny, the 20-acre linear park is located at what was once a thriving wharf area, and its design and layout are in keeping with its industrial past.

The park features 20 acres of indigenous landscaping, bike paths, playgrounds, a dog run, and the first of two multiuse pavilions transformed from former industrial wharves, including the Piety Wharf, which overlooks the Mississippi River and the New Orleans skyline and includes a garden and picnic area.

One of the park's signature features is the Piety Street Arch, a pedestrian footbridge that crosses active railroad tracks and the Mississippi River floodwall. Scheduled to open in late 2014 are the Mandeville Shed, an old industrial wharf being converted into an open-air event space; the Mandeville Ellipse, a raised grass lawn; and the Mandeville Crossing, which will feature stairs and elevators that connect to an elevated walkway leading to the riverfront.

Park hours are 8 a.m.–6 p.m., with hours extended to 7 p.m. during daylight-saving time. A public parking lot is located along Chartres Street at the foot of Piety Street.

The church is also home to the St. Gerard Community for the Deaf, which serves the spiritual needs of the area's deaf and hearing-impaired Catholics.

● Walk two blocks to the corner of Dauphine and Louisa Streets. On your stroll, take note of the sheer variety of houses, among them 19th- and 20th-century shotgun doubles, Creole cottages, and Craftsman bungalows, many of which have been transformed from dilapidated shacks to architectural masterpieces.

At the corner of Dauphine and Louisa, to your left, is Booty's Street Food, one of the myriad restaurants that opened in Bywater after Hurricane Katrina. If you're a "street-food geek," as Booty's calls its fans, you're sure to enjoy its global menu offerings, from *banh mi* (Vietnamese po'boys) and falafel sandwiches to empanadas and *yuca mofongo,* a Puerto Rican fritter stuffed with roast pork.

Across Dauphine is one of the newest entries in the Bywater culinary scene: Oxalis, a gastropub named for a plant that the owners noticed growing on the property opened in December 2013. It describes itself as a "whiskey-focused restaurant that just so happens to serve amazing food." The menu, designed to complement the extensive whiskey list, includes such items as Korean wings, cauliflower "steak," and sweet potato poutine.

A neighborhood like Bywater needs a good thrift store, so if you're in the market for secondhand stuff, check out the Bargain Center, at the opposite corner of Dauphine and Louisa. The place is packed to the gills with everything from antiques and jewelry to vintage photographs and Mexican folk art. The Bargain Center doesn't have much in the way of secondhand clothing, but the Pop Shop, next door at 3212 Dauphine, does.

- Continue walking in the 3200 block of Dauphine. At 3218 Dauphine is Satsuma Cafe, a cool eatery with an especially impressive selection of fresh-squeezed organic juices, from the Popeye (a mixture of spinach, lemon, kale, and apple) to the Cleanser (beet, fennel, cucumber, and lemon). The quinoa salad and the roasted-pear-and-brie melt are among the yummy items on the menu.

  At the end of the block on the left, at the corner of Dauphine and Piety, is Frady's One Stop Food Store, a convenience store that also makes a pretty decent po'boy, perfect for matching with a cold beer and enjoying at one of the outdoor tables.

- Turn right on Piety Street and walk one block to Royal Street past Mickey Markey Park, once a rundown playground that received a much-needed upgrade when city officials shut it down in 2011 because of high levels of lead contamination. In addition to remediation work, the park received fresh landscaping, updated playground equipment, and new concrete walkways.

- Walk one block to Chartres Street past Pizza Delicious, which got its start in 2010 as a twice-a-week pop-up. It proved so popular that when the owners decided to open a permanent eatery on Piety, they were able to raise some of their startup money through crowd sourcing. Pizza Delicious serves traditional New York–style pizza like cheese and pepperoni but also offers a special pizza of the day. Past pizza specials have included braised Brussels sprouts, wild boar and charred green onion sausage, and roasted cauliflower and marinated red onion. In 2013, Pizza Delicious made two national best-of lists: Its Hot Sopressata was named one of the website Thrillist's Top 33 Pizzas in America, and its plain cheese pizza was honored as one of The Daily Meal's 101 Best Pizzas in America.

Across the street from Pizza Delicious is Piety Street Sno-Balls, based at the Old Ironworks, which also hosts monthly flea markets, theatrical productions, festivals, and other events. Next to Pizza Delicious, in the hot-pink building at the corner of Piety and Chartres, is Euclid Records, which, in addition to selling new and used vinyl and CDs, stages live-music performances.

● Turn right on Chartres. Across the street is an arched staircase leading across railroad tracks to the new Crescent Park, a 1.4-mile linear green space that stretches from Elysian Fields Avenue in the Marigny to Mazant Street in Bywater (see sidebar). The park isn't included on this tour but is highly recommended.

● Walk one block and turn right on Louisa Street. Toward the end of the block, at 634 Louisa, is one of Bywater's most elegant homes, a late-19th-century raised center-hall Italianate cottage that houses The Country Club. Serving a largely gay clientele, The Country Club has a restaurant and bar inside and a swimming pool, cabana bar, and hot tub out back (the backyard amenities cost extra).

In contrast to the stateliness of The Country Club is Markey's Bar, a congenial dive that's been open since 1947. Markey's is a popular gathering spot for watching sports or trying one or two of the 25 beers on tap.

● Walk two blocks to the corner of Burgundy and Louisa. Maurepas Foods, at 3200 Burgundy, is another of the neighborhood's hip restaurants. The owners describe their menu as a "revolving door based on the available meats and produce of our purveyors." The fare includes dishes such as goat tacos, duck meatballs, and chorizo sandwiches.

● Walk two blocks to St. Claude Avenue, turn left, and walk one block to Clouet Street. At the corner of St. Claude and Clouet is Sugar Park, another pizza joint (try The Bird, topped with chicken Parmesan and lots of cheese). Across St. Claude is Saturn

Bar, another neighborhood dive that is consistently ranked as one of the top bars in New Orleans.

● Turn left on Clouet. Walk two blocks to Burgundy Street and turn right. Walk one block to Montegut, turn left, and return to the starting point at Montegut and Dauphine.

Although this is the end of the tour, there is so much more to Bywater, and we'd be remiss in not mentioning the neighborhood's other treasures—Elizabeth's, a down-home restaurant known for its praline bacon and fried green tomatoes; the music clubs Vaughn's and B. J.'s Lounge; and Bacchanal, a wine bar with a cool outdoor patio. For barbecue, try The Joint; for fried seafood, Jack Dempsey's.

POINTS OF INTEREST

Blessed Francis Xavier Seelos Catholic Church seeloschurchno.org, 3053 Dauphine St., 504-943-5566

Booty's Street Food bootysnola.com, 800 Louisa St., 504-266-2887

Oxalis oxalisbywater.com, 3162 Dauphine St., 504-267-4776

Bargain Center 3200 Dauphine St., 504-948-0007

Pop Shop 3212 Dauphine St. (no phone or website)

Satsuma Cafe satsumacafe.com, 3218 Dauphine St., 504-304-5962

Frady's One Stop Food Store 3231 Dauphine St., 504-949-9688

Mickey Markey Park 700 Piety St.

Pizza Delicious pizzadelicious.com, 617 Piety St., 504-676-8482

Piety Street Sno-Balls 612 Piety St., 504-782-2569

Euclid Records www.euclidnola.com, 3301 Chartres St., 504-947-4348

Crescent Park reinventingthecrescent.org, Mississippi Riverfront between Elysian Fields Avenue and Mazant Street, 504-658-4334

The Country Club thecountryclubneworleans.com, 634 Louisa St., 504-945-0742

Markey's Bar facebook.com/markeysbarnola, 640 Louisa St., 504-943-0785

Maurepas Foods maurepasfoods.com, 3200 Burgundy St., 504-267-0072

Sugar Park sugarparknola.com, 3054 St. Claude Ave., 504-942-2047

Saturn Bar saturnbar.com, 3067 St. Claude Ave., 504-949-7532

route summary

1. Begin at corner of Montegut and Dauphine Streets.
2. Walk three blocks to Piety Street and turn right.
3. Walk two blocks to Chartres Street and turn right.
4. Walk one block to Louisa Street and turn right.
5. Walk five blocks to St. Claude Avenue and turn left.
6. Walk one block to Clouet Street and turn left.
7. Walk two blocks to Burgundy Street and turn right.
8. Walk one block to Montegut Street, turn left, and return to starting point.

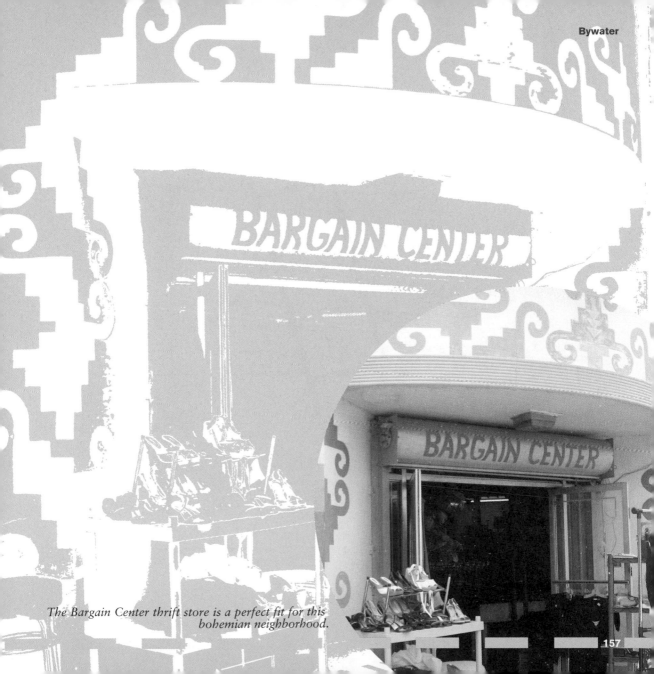

The Bargain Center thrift store is a perfect fit for this bohemian neighborhood.

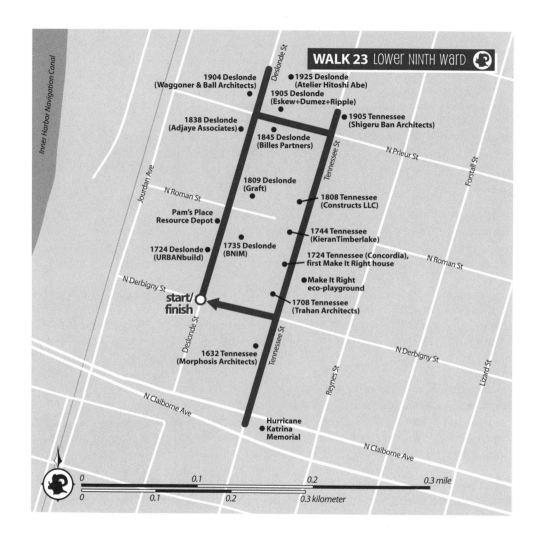

WALK 23 Lower Ninth Ward

1904 Deslonde
(Waggoner & Ball Architects)

1925 Deslonde
(Atelier Hitoshi Abe)

1905 Deslonde
(Eskew+Dumez+Ripple)

1838 Deslonde
(Adjaye Associates)

1905 Tennessee
(Shigeru Ban Architects)

1845 Deslonde
(Billes Partners)

N Prieur St

Jourdan Ave

N Roman St

1809 Deslonde
(Graft)

Tennessee St

Forstall St

1808 Tennessee
(Constructs LLC)

Pam's Place
Resource Depot

1744 Tennessee
(KieranTimberlake)

1724 Deslonde
(URBANbuild)

1735 Deslonde
(BNIM)

1724 Tennessee (Concordia),
first Make It Right house

N Roman St

N Derbigny St

Make It Right
eco-playground

start/
finish

1708 Tennessee
(Trahan Architects)

Deslonde St

Tennessee St

1632 Tennessee
(Morphosis Architects)

N Derbigny St

Reynes St

Lizard St

N Claiborne Ave

Hurricane
Katrina
Memorial

N Claiborne Ave

Inner Harbor Navigation Canal

0   0.1   0.2   0.3 mile

0   0.1   0.2   0.3 kilometer

23 LOWER NINTH WARD: MAKIN' IT RIGHT

BOUNDARIES: N. Claiborne Ave., Tennessee St., Deslonde St., N. Johnson St.
DISTANCE: 0.7 mile
PARKING: Free street parking
PUBLIC TRANSIT: It's best to drive to this neighborhood.

The Lower Ninth Ward of New Orleans, or the Lower Nine as locals call it, was one of the areas hardest hit by Hurricane Katrina, with multiple levee breaches flooding virtually the entire community. So powerful was the flood that it knocked houses off their foundations and killed hundreds of residents who were unable to escape.

While the majority of neighborhoods devastated by Katrina have recovered, the pace of rebuilding in the Lower Nine continues to drag nearly a decade after the storm. There are bright spots, however. Groups such as Habitat for Humanity and Common Ground Relief continue to lend their support to assist this mostly low-income part of New Orleans.

Another group making a difference is the Make It Right Foundation, a nonprofit endeavor that actor Brad Pitt established in 2007 to help bring residents back home. With architects from around the world lending their expertise, the group set out to construct 150 houses. But rather than build the new dwellings as they were, the group prioritized safety, sustainability, and of course, affordability.

The following walk is based on a self-guided tour recommended by Make It Right at **makeitright.org.** It comes with advice: When walking in this neighborhood, please respect the privacy of homeowners by walking on the sidewalk—not up driveways or through yards—and don't ask to go inside a particular house. Also, note that this continues to be an active construction site, so please don't enter a home that's still in the building phase.

● **Begin at 1724 Deslonde St. This home was built by students of the Tulane School of Architecture's URBANbuild program under the supervision of Byron Mouton, a Tulane professor of architecture and the house's designer. URBANbuild is a design-and-build program in which teams of students, working in partnership with a nonprofit** group such as Make It Right, take on the design and construction of prototypical homes for New Orleans neighborhoods.

- Continue to 1738 Deslonde, home of Pam's Place Resource Depot. Here you can learn about the effects of Katrina and the history of the Lower Ninth Ward and the Make It Right Foundation. You'll learn how the group builds its homes and what makes them energy-efficient, healthy, and safe for homeowners and the environment. For example, all homes are built with metal roofs, which absorb less heat, thereby reducing the cost of cooling a home. In addition, all homes are built at least 5 feet off the ground— 3 feet higher than federal standards—to protect them from Katrina-like flooding.

- Across the street at 1735 Deslonde is a house designed by BNIM of Kansas City, Missouri. The house was built in three modular parts and assembled on-site.

- Cross North Roman St. and continue walking to 1809 Deslonde. The yellow house to the right was built by Graft, a Berlin, Germany–based firm, in collaboration with Brad Pitt. The house is Graft's modern update to the traditional New Orleans shotgun.

- The house at 1838 Deslonde was designed by Adjaye Associates, a London-based company. The house uses the roof as a shaded terrace. Before building, architects met with the Lower Ninth Ward community, which stressed the importance of outdoor spaces and porches in home designs.

- On the right, at 1845 Deslonde, is a house that uses natural ventilation to keep it cool during the warm summer months. Designed by Billes Partners of New Orleans, it features high ceilings with fans and shading devices.

- Cross North Prieur Street and continue to 1905 Deslonde. This house, designed by Eskew+Dumez+Ripple of New Orleans, has large windows that allow for natural light in the communal rooms.

- At 1925 Deslonde is Make It Right's first duplex. Designed by Atelier Hitoshi Abe of Sendai, Japan, it features large open spaces that can be customized as private rooms and living areas.

- Turn around on Deslonde and walk to the house at 1904 Deslonde, designed by Waggoner & Ball Architects of New Orleans. Its design was inspired by the traditional camelback. A great room combines living and dining spaces, and there's outside exposure on three sides, allowing for nice views of the street and neighborhood.

- Turn left on North Prieur Street, then left again on Tennessee Street. At 1905 Tennessee is a home designed by Shigeru Ban Architects of Tokyo. This is the first Make It Right home with a green roof. Green roofs absorb rainwater, provide insulation, create a habitat for wildlife, and help cool houses in warm climates.

- Turn around on Tennessee and head in the opposite direction to 1808 Tennessee. This home, designed by Constructs LLC of Accra, Ghana, features an exterior stairway with a timber-framed roof designed to bring in light and keep out rain. The stairs are supported by steel rods, creating a floating effect.

- On the right, at 1744 Tennessee, is a home designed by KieranTimberlake of Philadelphia. The house has a roof deck, sunscreens, and a mesh trellis. The firm won the 2010 Committee on the Environment award from the American Institute of Architects for this design.

- At 1724 Tennessee is the first home completed by Make It Right in 2008, just three years after Katrina. It was designed by Concordia of New Orleans. Not long after this home and several others were built, Hurricane Gustav, a Category 3 storm, hit New Orleans. None of the Make It Right homes were damaged.

- On the left is the Make It Right eco-playground, a project of Kompan Inc., the Kellogg Company, and BNMI. The space is considered one of the most technically advanced eco-playgrounds in the country. The playground equipment is made of only sustainable and recyclable materials, including a solar-powered computer that allows children to play physically active digital games.

- At 1708 Tennessee Street is a house designed by Trahan Architects of Baton Rouge. Its rolling roof line provides shading on the south-facing side of the home and creates an outdoor space for the homeowner.

- Cross North Derbigny Street and continue walking on Tennessee. The house at 1632 Tennessee, to the right, can float in floodwaters of up to 16 feet. Designed by Morphosis Architects, it is held in place, in the event of a flood, by two steel guideposts. This is the first floating home permitted in the United States.

- Walk one block to North Claiborne Avenue and cross over to the neutral ground, where you'll see the Hurricane Katrina Memorial. The structure honors the victims of the storm and the spirit of survivors determined to rebuild their community.

- From the neutral ground, backtrack on Tennessee to North Claiborne and walk a block back up Tennessee. At North Derbigny, turn left and return to the starting point.

  Not included on this tour but just a few blocks away on Deslonde Street, the Lower Ninth Ward Living Museum features oral histories from community members, displays exhibits of key events in the history of the Lower Ninth Ward, and presents cultural events. It's best to drive here, though.

POINTS OF INTEREST

Hurricane Katrina Memorial North Claiborne Avenue between Tennessee and Reynes Streets
Lower Ninth Ward Living Museum l9livingmuseum.org, 1235 Deslonde St., 504-220-3652

ROUTE SUMMARY

1. Begin walk at North Derbigny and Deslonde Streets.
2. Walk three blocks to 1925 Deslonde and turn around.
3. Walk one block on Deslonde to North Prieur Street and turn left.
4. Walk one block to Tennessee Street and turn left.
5. Walk to 1905 Tennessee and turn around.
6. Walk three blocks to North Claiborne Avenue and cross to neutral ground.
7. Backtrack across North Claiborne and walk one block back up Tennessee to North Derbigny Street.
8. Turn left on North Derbigny to return to the starting point.

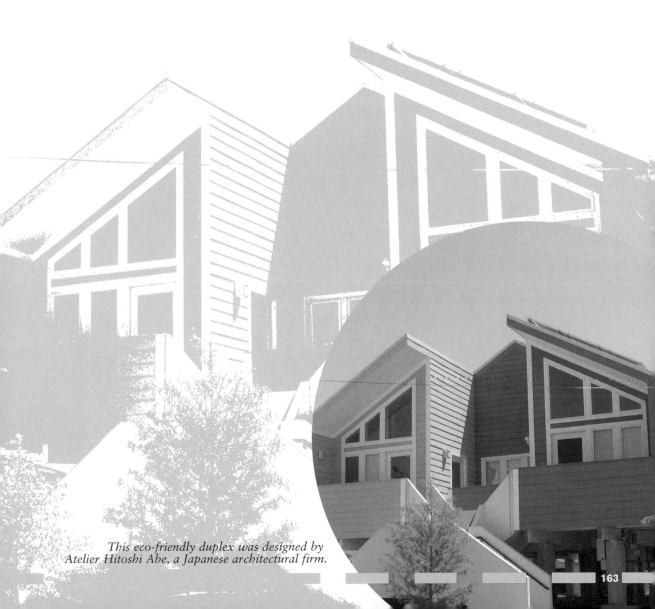

*This eco-friendly duplex was designed by
Atelier Hitoshi Abe, a Japanese architectural firm.*

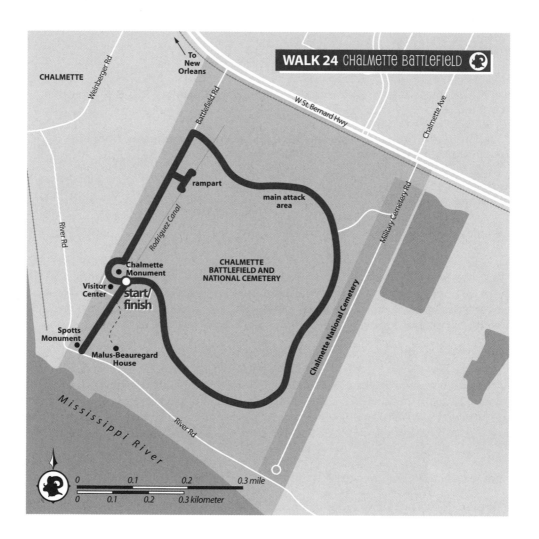

CHALMETTE

To New Orleans

WALK 24 CHALMETTE BATTLEFIELD

Weinberger Rd

Battlefield Rd

W St. Bernard Hwy

Chalmette Ave

River Rd

Rodriguez Canal

rampart

main attack area

Military Cemetery Rd

Chalmette Monument

CHALMETTE BATTLEFIELD AND NATIONAL CEMETERY

Visitor Center

start/ finish

Chalmette National Cemetery

Spotts Monument

Malus-Beauregard House

Mississippi River

River Rd

0   0.1   0.2   0.3 mile
0   0.1   0.2   0.3 kilometer

24 CHALMETTE BATTLEFIELD: WHERE WAR WAS WAGED

BOUNDARIES: St. Bernard Hwy., Mississippi River, Military Cemetery Rd., Battlefield Rd.
DISTANCE: 2 miles
PARKING: At the Visitor Center
PUBLIC TRANSIT: None, but the paddlewheeler *Creole Queen* travels here from the French Quarter. Visit creolequeen.com for more information.

As you drive down St. Bernard Highway, an industrial stretch of road dotted with oil refineries and chemical companies, it seems almost inconceivable that a decisive battle in the War of 1812 was fought just behind the Norfolk-Southern Railroad tracks in St. Bernard Parish, about 7 miles from downtown New Orleans.

The day was January 8, 1815, and Maj. Gen. Andrew Jackson's stunning victory over experienced British troops—in less than 2 hours—was considered the greatest American land victory of the War of 1812. The Battle of New Orleans not only preserved America's claim to the Louisiana Territory, it led to migration and settlement along the Mississippi River and made Jackson, who would go on to become the seventh president of the United States, a national hero.

One of six sites in Jean Lafitte National Historical Park and Preserve, Chalmette Battlefield tells the story of the war through exhibits and films at the Visitor Center, along with a 1.5-mile walk around the grounds and various other outdoor exhibits. Every January, the park brings the past to life with a living-history celebration featuring cannon and musket firings, period crafts and cooking, War of 1812 military drills and tactics, war reenactments, and an evening lantern tour. In January 2015, the battlefield celebrated its bicentennial with four days of activities.

Like other historical sites in and around New Orleans, this one is reputed to harbor spirits: Many paranormal experts consider Chalmette one of the most haunted battlefields in the US.

A few tips: Steer clear of small mounds of dirt, where fire ants may live. Don't climb the oak trees in the picnic area. Don't bring metal detectors on park property—relic hunting is strictly forbidden. And as you're walking, be on the lookout for cars, because this walk covers the same ground as the park's self-guided driving tour.

- Begin at the Visitor Center, where you can learn about the importance of the Battle of New Orleans in the War of 1812 through displays, maps, interactive exhibits and films. The center's museum store sells books, period music, reproductions of war memorabilia, and children's books. Chalmette Battlefield sustained major damage in Hurricane Katrina; the visitor center was destroyed, and most of the structures were damaged. Although the battlefield reopened a year after the storm—in September 2006—it didn't fully recover until 2010, when the new Visitor Center was completed.

- After exiting the Visitor Center, head a few feet to the left to Battlefield Tour Loop Road, a 1.5-mile roadway with stations where you can sit on a bench and read plaques that explain the war's major milestones. As you begin walking, look to your right at the Malus-Beauregard House, a restored Greek Revival mansion built nearly 20 years after the Battle of New Orleans. The house is named after its first and last owners—Madeleine Pannetier Malus in the 1830s and Judge René Beauregard (son of Confederate general P. G. T. Beauregard) in 1880. The National Park Service, which runs Chalmette Battlefield, bought the house in 1949.

- Continue walking around the loop where you'll pass exhibits that explain the British battle plan, which called for attacks along the river, against the American rampart near the swamp, and on the west bank. Other exhibits explain the British artillery batteries, the roads and ditches used for the assault, and the march of the 93rd Highlanders across the battlefield. (The American line of defense is explained on the walkway leading into the park.)

- At around the halfway point, you'll see a pathway leading to Chalmette National Cemetery. It's not included in this walk, but feel free to explore the grounds where more than 15,000 war veterans are buried. The cemetery was established in May 1864 as a final resting place for Union soldiers who died in Louisiana during the Civil War. The cemetery also includes the gravesites of veterans of the Spanish-American War, World Wars I and II, and the Vietnam War. Four Americans who fought in the War of 1812 are also buried in the cemetery, though only one of them took part in the Battle of New Orleans.

- From the cemetery, continue circling around the loop to the area that served as the main attack of the British under Maj. Gen. Edward M. Pakenham, commander of the

British army at Chalmette, and Maj. Gen. Samuel Gibbs. On January 8, 1815, Pakenham sent 7,000 troops head-on against the American position, concentrating their attack on the rampart's ends. But the American troops responded with devastating effect. Pakenham, Gibbs, and other high-ranking officers were killed or wounded, and the British soon surrendered.

● Turn left on Battlefield Road, heading south and west. The story of the American line of defense is told in exhibits that run along the rampart and Rodriguez Canal. The exhibits describe American troops, their weapons, the 1815 landscape, and the last major battle of the War of 1812.

● Circle past the west side of the Chalmette Monument, then head straight past the Visitor Center and take the path to the left. You'll come to a three-way intersection—take the path that forks right to the Spotts Monument, erected in honor of Maj. Samuel Spotts, who fired the first gun in the Battle of New Orleans. Between the Malus-Beauregard House (to your left) and the river (straight ahead), you'll see exhibits telling the stories of the land and the people who lived here after the battle, including the development of a thriving free African American community.

● At the end of the walkway, turn around and follow it back to the three-way intersection; then make a quick right, followed by a quick left, to reach the Chalmette Monument. Walk around the 100-foot-tall obelisk, which pays homage to the troops of the Battle of New Orleans. The cornerstone honoring the American victory at New Orleans was laid in January 1840, within days after Andrew Jackson visited the field on the battle's

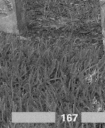

Take some time to stroll through Chalmette National Cemetery, where more than 15,000 war veterans are buried.

25th anniversary. The state of Louisiana began building the monument in 1855, and it was completed in 1908. If you're up to it, consider climbing its 122 interior steps to the viewing platform at the top. If you do, take your time—while the climb isn't overly strenuous, the steps and handrails may be slick in wet or humid weather. Children should be accompanied by an adult.

POINTS OF INTEREST

Chalmette Battlefield and National Cemetery nps.gov/jela/chalmette-battlefield.htm, 8606 W. St. Bernard Highway, Chalmette; 504-281-0510

ROUTE SUMMARY

1.   Beginning at the Visitor Center, follow Battlefield Tour Loop Road counterclockwise around the battlefield to Battlefield Road, and turn left.

2.   Follow Battlefield Road southwest; then circle right around the west side of the Chalmette Monument, head straight past the Visitor Center, and turn left.

3   At the three-way junction, bear right on the walkway leading to the Spotts Monument.

4   Turn around and head back to the three-way junction.

5.   Make a quick right, then a quick left, to reach the Chalmette Monument.

6.   Circle the monument and end at the Visitor Center.

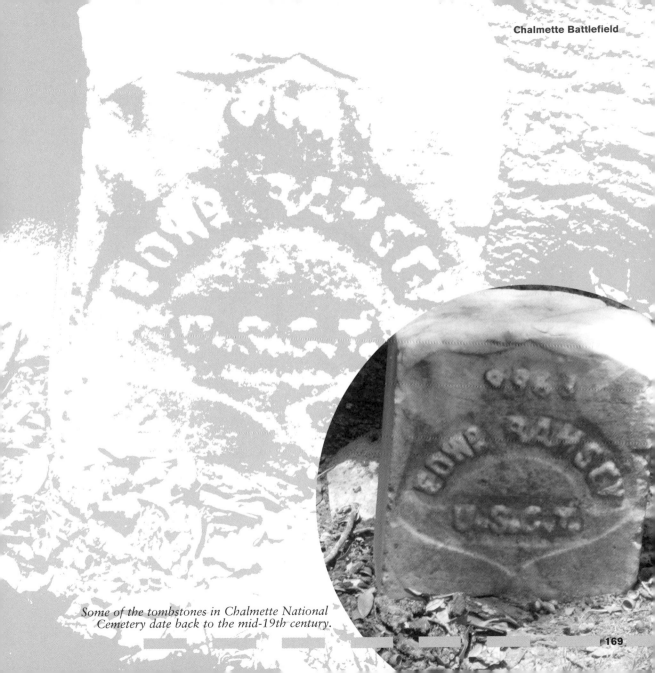

*Some of the tombstones in Chalmette National
Cemetery date back to the mid-19th century.*

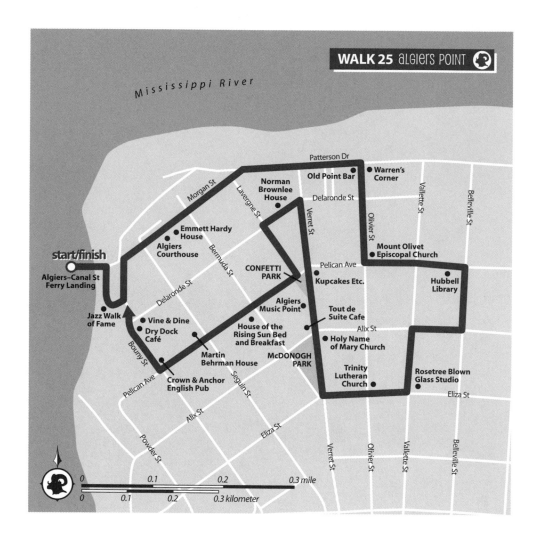

Mississippi River

Patterson Dr

● Warren's
Corner

Old Point Bar ●

Morgan St

Lavergne St

Norman
Brownlee
House

Delaronde St

Verret St

Vallette St

Belleville St

Olivier St

**Emmett Hardy
House** ●

Algiers
Courthouse ●

Bermuda St

**Mount Olivet
Episcopal Church** ●

start/finish
○

**Algiers–Canal St
Ferry Landing**

**CONFETTI
PARK**

Pelican Ave

**Hubbell
Library**

Delaronde St

Kupcakes Etc. ●

**Jazz Walk
of Fame** ●

Algiers
Music Point ●

**Tout de
Suite Cafe** ●

● **Vine & Dine**
● **Dry Dock
Café**

**House of the
Rising Sun Bed
and Breakfast**

Alix St

Bouny St

**Martin
Behrman House**

**McDONOGH
PARK**

● **Holy Name
of Mary Church**

**Rosetree Blown
Glass Studio** ●

Pelican Ave

**Crown & Anchor
English Pub** ●

Segulin St

**Trinity
Lutheran
Church** ●

Eliza St

Alix St

Eliza St

Powder St

Verret St

Olivier St

Vallette St

Belleville St

0   0.1   0.2   0.3 mile
0   0.1   0.2   0.3 kilometer

25 ALGIERS POINT: BEST OF THE WEST BANK

BOUNDARIES: Morgan St./Patterson Dr., Belleville St., Eliza St.
DISTANCE: 1.5 miles
PARKING: Free on the street, but check signs for time limits.
PUBLIC TRANSIT: Algiers–Canal Street ferry

Algiers Point is one of those "best kept secret" kinds of neighborhoods—one that mixes the charm and character of Uptown New Orleans with the affordability and quaintness of small-town America. For some house hunters, its location on the West Bank of the Mississippi River is an immediate turnoff. For others, it's the perfect landing spot.

Typically referred to as "The Point," Algiers Point is nestled within Algiers, the only part of New Orleans located on the West Bank. Listed on the National Register of Historic Places, it is the second oldest neighborhood in New Orleans—the French Quarter is first—and while most of it was destroyed in the Great Fire of 1895, its rebuilt residences, from Creole cottages to Greek Revivals, give it the feel of a 19th-century village.

One of Algiers Point's biggest draws is the Algiers–Canal Street ferry, which runs all day long and can carry pedestrians and bicyclists to either side of the river in a matter of minutes. Residents often boast that they can get to downtown New Orleans more quickly than many who live on the East Bank.

The Point is also home to a number of locally owned restaurants; music clubs and cafés; and, over the past few years, music festivals, art and farmers' markets, home tours, and other events have attracted locals and visitors alike.

● **Begin at the Algiers–Canal Street ferry landing.** If you've taken the ferry from downtown New Orleans, you've already noticed the spectacular view of the city's skyline. If you've traveled by car, walk to the top of the levee and take in its beauty. Also at the top of the levee is the Jazz Walk of Fame, a project of the New Orleans Jazz National Historic Park. The paved walkway features tributes to such jazz greats as Louis Armstrong, Jelly Roll Martin, and Al Hirt. Jazz plays an important role in the history of

Algiers Point, with countless musicians having made their homes in this West Bank community. A free audio tour is available by calling 504-613-4062.

- Take the stairs or ramp down to ground level. The Dry Dock Café, to the right, is an Algiers Point institution that offers a great selection of local brews, po'boys, and burgers. Next to the Dry Dock is Vine & Dine, a wine bar and gourmet pizzeria.

- Turn left on Morgan Street, which turns into Patterson Drive (also known as the River Road). Check out the Algiers Courthouse, a Romanesque-style structure built in 1896 after the previous courthouse burned in the 1895 blaze. The courthouse houses a small-claims court, voter-registration and marriage-license offices, and other services. Behind the courthouse is a carriage house that was once home to a stable and jail. The Friends of the Algiers Courthouse assists the city of New Orleans in preserving and maintaining the property. Every spring, the group holds a crawfish-boil fundraiser to help in its preservation efforts.

- Two doors from the courthouse, at 237 Morgan St., is the former home of jazz musician Emmett Hardy, a cornetist who died in 1925. Hardy played in Brownlee's Orchestra; the New Orleans Rhythm Kings; and with violinist Oscar Marcour, the Boswell Sisters, and drummer Arthur "Monk" Hazel. Hardy lived in the house from 1920 to 1923.

- Continue walking down Morgan Street. The tall red building to the left is a luxury-condominium development, one of the few modern structures to be built on the Point.

- Walk three blocks to the corner of Patterson Drive and Olivier Street. The Old Point Bar is a haven for music lovers, with live performances almost every night. The bar features outdoor seating, pool tables and dart boards, and local brews. Across the street is Warren's Corner, a one-time Cajun restaurant now used as a special-events venue and an occasional film set.

- At the Old Point Bar, turn right on Olivier Street and walk two blocks to Pelican Avenue, past beautifully landscaped and brightly painted homes, many designed in the Greek Revival style. At the corner of Olivier and Pelican is Mount Olivet Episcopal Church. Founded in 1845, it is built entirely of cypress and, according to the church, has withstood several fires and hurricanes.

● Turn left on Pelican Avenue. The Hubbell Library, at 725 Pelican, is New Orleans's oldest public library, having been built in 1907 with a donation from Andrew Carnegie. The library has seen its share of hard times, most notably in the 1960s when roof leaks, falling plaster, and buckling floors forced it to close. Because the city was building a new, more modern library in another part of Algiers about 4 miles away, officials decided to shut down the Algiers Point branch, much to the disappointment of neighborhood residents. It reopened in 1975 following a grassroots campaign led by resident and activist Cita Dennis Hubbell, who cited the building's architecture, history, and neighborhood convenience as reasons to save it. Hubbell had such an impact on the library's survival that it was renamed in her memory after she died in 2002.

Although the building escaped serious damage after Hurricane Katrina—it reopened after a couple of months—structural problems predating the storm shut it down again in 2008. The library operated out of a temporary branch at the Carriage House behind the Algiers Courthouse, where it remained until July 2013, when a repaired Hubbell Library reopened for the third time.

● Walk to the corner of Pelican and Belleville Street, where you'll see Belleville Assisted Living, a retirement community built on the site of the old Belleville School, which dates back to 1895. Turn right on Belleville, walk one block to Alix Street, turn right, and walk one block to Vallette Street.

● Turn left on Vallette Street and walk one block to the Rosetree Blown Glass Studio and Gallery, at the corner of Vallette and Eliza Streets. Housed in the old Algy Theater, which has maintained its Art Deco look, the studio creates exquisite works of art— from perfume bottles to vases—using traditional glassblowing techniques. The gallery offers a viewing window where visitors can watch the artists at work.

● Turn right and walk two blocks on Eliza Street to Verret Street, past Trinity Lutheran Church on your right. Dating back to the mid-1870s, the church was organized by a group of German families in Algiers. The congregation's first house of worship was dedicated in 1876, the current Gothic/Colonial Revival–style church in 1911.

● Turn right on Verret Street and walk one block to Alix Street, passing McDonogh Park—also known as the Bermuda Triangle because it's bounded by Bermuda, Verret, and Alix Streets—on your left. In April 2013, the park received a long-awaited make-over, with volunteers painting signs, building wooden benches, and installing a new baseball diamond. The green space is also home to the Algiers War Memorial.

At the corner of Verret and Alix is Holy Name of Mary Church, which was built in 1929 in the Tudor Gothic style. The church has more than 75 stained-glass windows and marble and artwork from a previous church building.

- Continue on Verret past the Tout de Suite Cafe, an adorable eatery that's open for breakfast and lunch. About a half-block down is Algiers Music Point, which sells an array of musical instruments, including vintage guitars. Just past the music shop, at Verret Street and Pelican Avenue, is Confetti Park, a haven for the pint-size set. This pocket park has playground equipment and picnic tables under cypress trees, plus a fence with confetti-like cutouts. In 2000, residents joined together to form Confetti Kids, a nonprofit group that holds family-friendly events such as an Easter-egg hunt, a Spooktacular Halloween Party, and a Friendship Day Parade. The group's signature event is the Candy Land Ball and Fundraiser.

- Continue on Verret. Just to the left, at Pelican and Verret, is what was once one of the longest-operating service stations in the South. For many years, it was home to Gulf Pizza, a tiny but beloved pizza joint; the owners closed shop in 2014, and as of this writing it was unclear if another restaurant would take over the site. On the opposite corner, facing Pelican Avenue, is Kupcakes Etc., where daily cupcake favorites include red velvet, ice-cream sundae, pecan praline, and coconut pleasure.

- Continue on Verret to Delaronde Street and turn left. The house at 407 Delaronde is the one-time residence of jazz musician Norman Brownlee, a pianist and bandleader who died in 1967 and who lived at this address from 1912 to 1922. He was the leader of Brownlee's Orchestra, which also featured Emmett Hardy and Arthur "Monk" Hazel, among other musicians.

- Walk one block to Lavergne Street and turn left; then walk one block to Pelican and turn right. A little more than a block ahead on your left, at 335 Pelican after you cross Bermuda Street, is House of the Rising Sun Bed and Breakfast, which the owners named after the fictitious house of ill repute that The Animals made famous in their

1964 hit song. The house was built in 1896 after the original 1870 cottage burned down in the Great Fire of 1895.

● Cross Seguin Street. In the next block, on your right at 228 Pelican, is the one-time home of Mayor Martin Behrman, who served as New Orleans's leader for four consecutive terms from 1904 to 1920. He served again from 1925 to 1926, when he died in office at age 61. Today, there are streets, schools, and parks named after Behrman.

At the end of the block, on the corner of Pelican and Bouny Street, is the Crown & Anchor, a British-style watering hole known for its Thursday-night pub quizzes, dart games, and an impressive selection of draft and bottled beers.

● Turn right on Bouny and walk two blocks back to the ferry landing.

POINTS OF INTEREST

Jazz Walk of Fame nps.gov/jazz, Algiers–Canal Street Ferry Terminal, 504-589-4841

Dry Dock Café thedrydockcafe.com, 133 Delaronde St., 504-361-8240

Vine & Dine vine-dine.com, 141 Delaronde St., 504-361-1402

Algiers Courthouse friendsofalgierscourthouse.org, 225 Morgan St.

Old Point Bar 545 Patterson Drive, 504-364-0950

Mount Olivet Episcopal Church mountolivet.org, 530 Pelican Ave., 504-366-4650

Cita Dennis Hubbell Library hubbelllibrary.org, 725 Pelican Ave., 504-596-3113

Rosetree Blown Glass Studio rosetreegallery.com, 446 Vallette St., 888-767-8733

Trinity Lutheran Church sites.google.com/site/trinityalgierspoint, 620 Eliza St., 504-368-0411

McDonogh Park Bounded by Bermuda, Verret, and Alix Streets

Tout de Suite Cafe toutdesuitecafe.com, 347 Verret St., 504-362-2264

Algiers Music Point algiersmusicpoint.com, 323 Verret St., 504-304-4201

Confetti Park 451 Pelican Ave. at Verret Street

Kupcakes Etc. kupcakesetc.angelfire.com, 501 Pelican Ave., 504-364-9384

House of the Rising Sun Bed and Breakfast risingsunbnb.com, 335 Pelican Ave.,
    504-231-6498

Crown & Anchor English Pub crownanchorpub.com, 200 Pelican Ave., 504-227-1007

route summary

1. From ferry landing, turn left on Morgan Street, which turns into Patterson Drive, and walk five blocks to Olivier Street.

2. Turn right on Olivier and walk two blocks to Pelican Avenue.

3. Turn left on Pelican and walk two blocks to Belleville Street.

4. Turn right on Belleville and walk one block to Alix Street.

5. Turn right on Alix and walk one block to Vallette Street.

6. Turn left on Vallette and walk one block to Eliza Street.

7. Turn right on Eliza and walk two blocks to Verret Street.

8. Turn right on Verret and walk three blocks to Delaronde Street.

9. Turn left on Delaronde and walk one block to Lavergne Street.

10. Turn left on Lavergne and walk one block to Pelican.

11. Turn right on Pelican and walk three blocks to Bouny Street.

12. Turn right on Bouny and walk two blocks back to ferry landing.

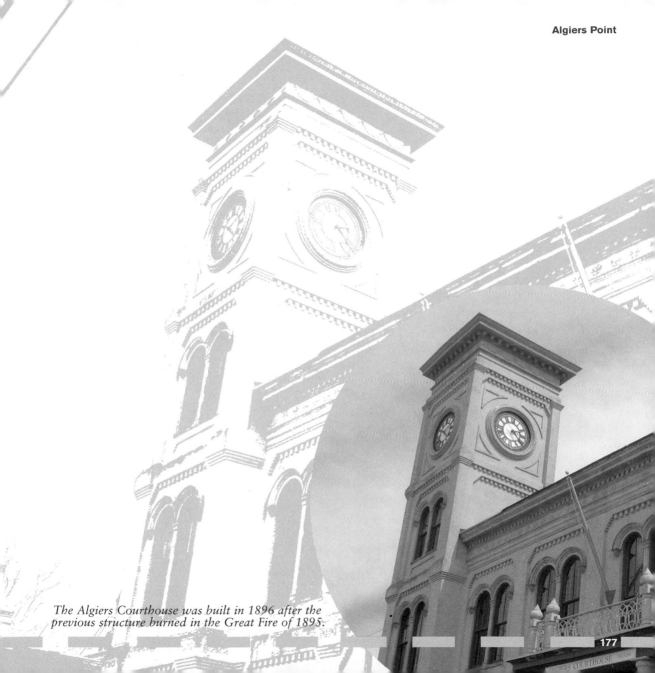

The Algiers Courthouse was built in 1896 after the previous structure burned in the Great Fire of 1895.

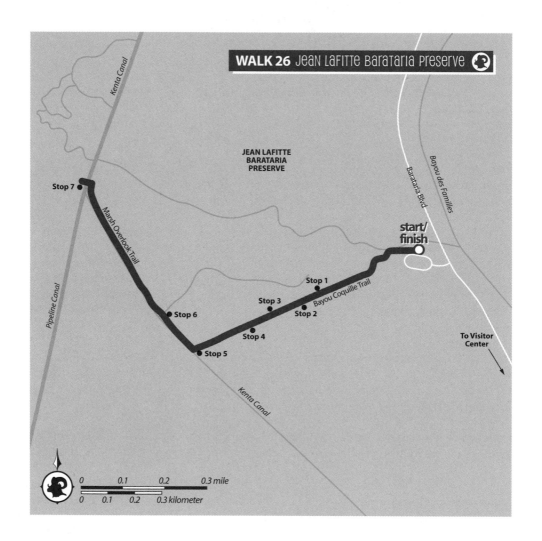

WALK 26 Jean Lafitte Barataria Preserve

Kenta Canal

JEAN LAFITTE
BARATARIA
PRESERVE

Barataria Blvd

Bayou des Familles

Marsh Overlook Trail

Pipeline Canal

Stop 7

start/
finish

Stop 1

Stop 3

Bayou Coquille Trail

Stop 2

Stop 6

Stop 4

Stop 5

Kenta Canal

To Visitor
Center

0   0.1   0.2   0.3 mile

0   0.1   0.2   0.3 kilometer

26 Jean Lafitte Barataria Preserve: Wetlands Wonder

BOUNDARIES: Not applicable—this is an out-and-back walk on two trails within the preserve.
DISTANCE: 1.8 miles
PARKING: Free parking at trailhead
PUBLIC TRANSIT: None

You won't find swings, golf courses, or amusement park rides at Jean Lafitte National Historical Park's Barataria Preserve, but what you will find is one of the most stunning displays of nature that Louisiana has to offer.

With 23,000 acres of swamp, marsh, trails, and waterways, Barataria Preserve is a park like no other. On the West Bank of Jefferson Parish, about 20 miles from downtown New Orleans, it offers an up-close encounter with some of the state's endangered wetlands amid a setting of live oaks, bald cypress, palmettos, and wildflowers. Walk on any of the preserve's boardwalk or gravel trails, and you'll likely see a variety of wildlife from alligators and snakes to armadillos and nutria, not to mention more than 200 species of birds, among them pelicans and bald eagles.

That's not to say the park doesn't have its challenges. Hurricane Katrina destroyed or damaged 60 percent of the preserve's biggest trees, resulting in more light for invasive non-native plants. The park's famous springtime iris blooms were especially affected, but the exquisite purple flowers are beginning to make a comeback.

The trails we've chosen are the Bayou Coquille Trail and the Marsh Overlook Trail, both of which are wheelchair-accessible and only about a mile from the Visitor Center. Be sure to stop at the center before you begin your hike. The center features dioramas, exhibits, a video, and hands-on display. Park rangers are on hand to answer any questions you might have. In addition, the walk has seven stops, where you can phone 504-799-0802 to get an audio description of each one. (The following descriptions are based on the audio tour.)

Some tips to keep in mind before you begin: Stay on boardwalks and trails, don't bring food or try to feed animals, don't pick flowers or dig up plants, and leave your pets at home. If you're taking the walk during the summer, bring a hat, insect repellent, and bottled water. And don't forget your camera and binoculars.

- **Access the Bayou Coquille Trail from the Bayou Coquille parking lot, about a mile from the Visitor Center. The park recommends this trail to first-time visitors because it is one of the preserve's most diverse. It begins on high ground deposited by flooding from Bayou des Familles, once a major distributary of the Mississippi River. Dating back 2,000 years, it was once an American Indian village. The trail will take you through hardwood forest with live oaks, dwarf palmettos, bald cypress, and the freshwater marsh's floating prairie of grasses and aquatic plants.**

- **Walk to Stop 1, where you'll be facing Bayou Coquille. *Coquille* is French for "shell," and the bayou got its name from the mounds of clamshells found here by early French surveyors. The discarded shells are evidence of a prehistoric Indian settlement, where Native Americans would consume small clams to supplement their diets of game, fish, and plants.**

- **Walk to Stop 2 and take note of the live oaks. Live oaks are the densest, strongest wood native to North America. In the late 1700s and early 1800s, oak lumber was used to build war ships. Live oaks typically grow thick trunks and wide-spreading limbs, and their low centers of gravity and extensive root systems help them resist high winds and storms. The trees at Barataria Preserve are 250–400 years old and are reasonably healthy, though many have lost limbs in hurricanes or have been struck by lightning. Notice the resurrection ferns on the tree branches. In dry weather, they curl and turn brown. When it rains, the leaves unfurl and turn green.**

- **Walk to Stop 3, where you'll learn the story of lumbering in Barataria from the 1880s to the 1920s. Loggers were especially attracted to bald cypress like the one in front of you. Bald cypress, which can grow up to 100 feet high and 15 feet in diameter, are resistant to rot and extremely durable. The logging process was grueling: Loggers would cut the huge trees by hand with crosscut saws, all while standing in mud and water and dealing with the threat of insects and snakes. Cables were then attached** to the logs and dragged to the end of the canal, where they were bound together to make rafts, which then floated to the sawmill.

- Walk to Stop 4, where you'll see a variety of invasive species of plants in the water below you, such as alligator weed, water hyacinth, and floating ferns called salvinia. They're called invasive because they are not native to Louisiana, having been brought by travelers from South America and Asia who did not realize the new plants would be destructive to the local environment. The invasive species have taken the place of native species such as wild iris and duckweed. Nutria, large rodents that call the preserve home, are also invasive species. They were brought to Louisiana in the 1930s for fur farming, replacing the native muskrats. The National Park Service has a program that aims to limit the growth of nonnative plant and animal species, but park rangers say it's impossible to eliminate them completely.

- Walk to Stop 5, where you'll learn the important story of Louisiana's wetlands. Look across the canal to open marsh. Park officials say that if you return here in a few years, some of the marshland may be gone. Surges from tropical storms and hurricanes destroy vegetation, and rebuilding land or at least slowing the rate of the land's disappearance is a massive project.

- Walk to Stop 6. One of the thrills of the Barataria Preserve trails is spotting alligators in the swamps. There's a healthy population of gators here, though some may be harder to spot than others. Although they can grow to up to 16 feet long, the longest alligators here are about 13 feet long. Alligators, along with the swamp's other animals and plants, are protected by law.

Alligators abound in the swamps of Jean Lafitte Barataria Preserve.
Photo: Donna Goldenberg

- At the half-mile point, you'll enter the Marsh Overlook Trail, which is situated atop a bank that was formed by dredged material from the Kenta Canal. Once used for irrigating and draining plantation fields, the canal was deepened and widened in the late 19th century so loggers could gain access to the bald-cypress swamp.

- Walk to Stop 7, where you'll learn that the grassland in the distance is actually a freshwater marsh that is not connected to the soil but is rather a floating mat of plants called a flotant. The marsh rises and falls with the water beneath it and is especially affected by wind direction and rainfall. Among the wildlife that call the flotant home are rabbits, alligators, raccoons, nutria, coyotes, whitetail deer, and many species of birds.

- Turn around at the end of the Marsh Outlook Trail and make your way back to the beginning of the Bayou Coquille Trail. If you're up to it, check out some of the park's other trails, or save them for your next visit.

POINTS OF INTEREST

Barataria Preserve, Jean Lafitte National Historical Park nps.gov/jela/barataria-preserve.htm, 6588 Barataria Blvd., Marrero; 504-689-3690, Ext. 10

ROUTE SUMMARY

1. Begin at entrance of Bayou Coquille Trail.
2. Walk a half-mile to Marsh Overlook Trail.
3. Walk another 0.4 mile to end of trail.
4. Turn around and return to starting point.

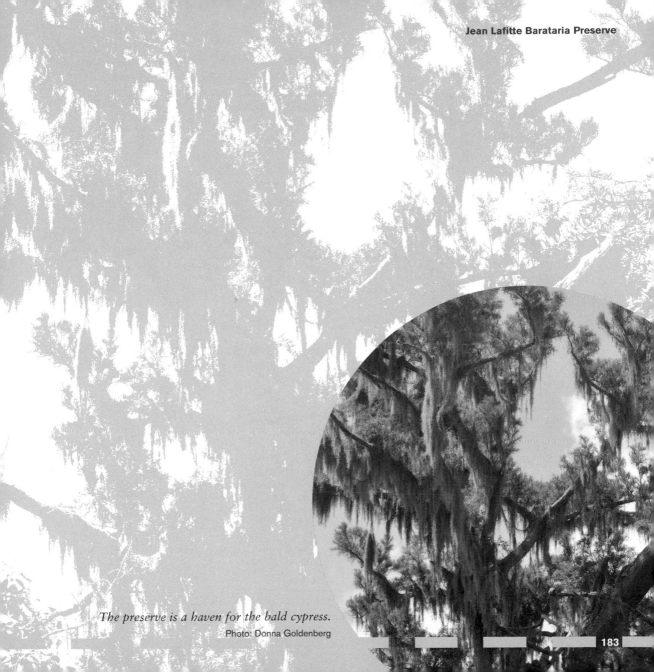

The preserve is a haven for the bald cypress.
Photo: Donna Goldenberg

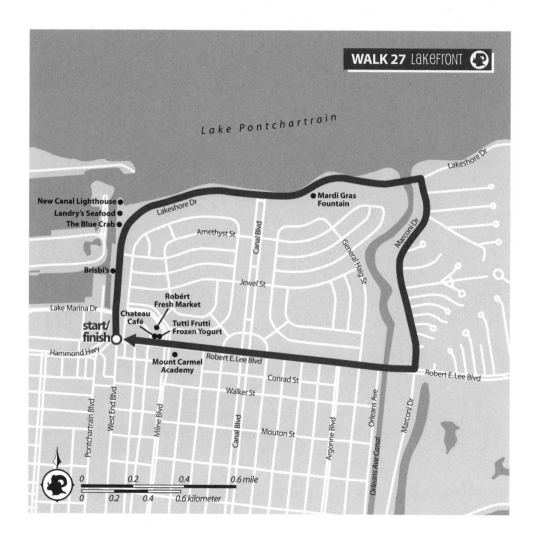

Lake Pontchartrain

New Canal Lighthouse ●
Landry's Seafood ●
The Blue Crab ●

Lakeshore Dr

● Mardi Gras
Fountain

Lakeshore Dr

Amethyst St

Canal Blvd

General Haig St

Marconi Dr

Brisbi's ●

Jewel St

Lake Marina Dr

Robért
Fresh Market

Chateau
Café

start/
finish

Tutti Frutti
Frozen Yogurt

Hammond Hwy

Mount Carmel
Academy

Robert E. Lee Blvd

Robert E. Lee Blvd

Conrad St

Pontchartrain Blvd

West End Blvd

Milne Blvd

Walker St

Canal Blvd

Mouton St

Argonne Blvd

Orleans Ave

Orleans Ave Canal

Marconi Dr

0   0.2   0.4   0.6 mile
0   0.2   0.4   0.6 kilometer

27 Lakefront: It's a Breeze

BOUNDARIES: **Robert E. Lee Blvd., Lakeshore Dr., Marconi Dr.**
DISTANCE: **3.1 miles**
PARKING: **Free parking on Robert E. Lee, in surrounding neighborhood, and at shopping-center parking lot**
PUBLIC TRANSIT: **RTA Bus #45 (Lakeview)**

The Lakefront area may not hold the popularity of the Garden District or the French Quarter, but avid walkers consider it one of the most refreshing and invigorating places to take a stroll. That is especially true of Lakeshore Drive, which meanders several miles along Lake Pontchartrain, the Crescent City's most expansive body of water and a sort of home-away-from-home for local boating enthusiasts.

Lake Pontchartrain covers a 630-square-foot area, has an average depth of 14–16 feet, and touches six different parishes (counties). The lake is part of the Lake Pontchartrain Basin, which comprises numerous bodies of water that connect to the Gulf of Mexico through the Mississippi River.

Over the years, the lake has seen its share of environmental challenges, among them urban runoff, saltwater intrusion, and wetlands loss. In 1989, the nonprofit Lake Pontchartrain Basin Foundation was established to essentially save the lake. Its efforts have and continue to pay off. Seasonal swimming is allowed in designated areas, and water quality is monitored and publicized weekly at **saveourlake.org.**

Every year, the foundation sponsors a number of events, with proceeds going toward its various preservation and educational programs. Some include the Back to the Beach Festival and the Save Our Lake and Coast Fishing Rodeo. Every September, volunteer groups come together for the annual Beach Sweep, a massive cleanup effort.

● **Start at the intersection of Lakeshore Drive and Robert E. Lee Boulevard. Stay on the east side of Lakeshore and head north toward the lake. About a block down is Lake Marina Drive, where the Orleans Marina is located. Lake Marina Drive leads to West End Park, a 30-acre green space around which sits the Southern Yacht Club** and the New Orleans Municipal Yacht Harbor. For years, West End Park was home to a bustling seafood restaurant industry, but a series of storms and hurricanes over the years—including Katrina—wiped it out.

- Continue walking along Lakeshore Drive past several restaurants to your left. Brisbi's and The Blue Crab opened in 2013, both as a dream by their owners to bring waterfront dining back to the neighborhood. Landry's has been around longer, its views of Lake Pontchartrain simply breathtaking.

  As Lakeshore bends to the right, you'll see Louisiana's only working lighthouse. In 2005, the lighthouse was severely damaged in Hurricanes Katrina and Rita but the Lake Pontchartrain Basin Foundation has since rebuilt and transformed it into the New Canal Lighthouse Museum and Education Center. The center offers programs on the history of the lighthouse, the ecology of the Pontchartrain Basin, and the critical coastal issues facing South Louisiana.

- Continue walk along Lakeshore Drive. To the right is the lakefront park, which, with its playgrounds, picnic shelters, and picnic pavilions, is the ideal place to spend a lazy weekend afternoon. Feel free to cross Lakeshore and get a closer view of the lake. But be extra-cautious, because this is a busy street.

  One of the highlights of the walk—besides the lake itself—is the famed Mardi Gras Fountain, between Canal Boulevard and Marconi Drive. Like the Lighthouse, the fountain sustained severe damage in Katrina but is now back to its original splendor. First built in 1960, the fountain is surrounded by plaques depicting the crests of Carnival organizations and krewes, including Rex, Bacchus, and Endymion.

- Continue walking on Lakeshore, cross the Orleans Avenue Canal, and turn right on Marconi Drive. Walk down the steps on the left side of the street. You are now in the Lake Vista subdivision, which, along with West and East Lakeshore and Lake Terrace, makes up the lakefront's residential area. Lake Vista is the most interesting of the three areas, its design based on the Garden City movement under which all interior streets end in culs-de-sac and separate pedestrian lanes meet at the center of the development.

- Walk eight blocks to Robert E. Lee Boulevard. Notice that the streets of Lake Vista are named for birds, such as Hawk and Swan, and the lanes for flowers, such as Azalea and Daisy. The neighborhood sustained substantial damage in Katrina, and many homes were rebuilt higher and sturdier.

- At Robert E. Lee, turn right and continue walking over the Orleans Avenue Canal toward Canal Boulevard. Cross Canal and walk back to your starting point, just past Mount Carmel Academy, one of the city's oldest and most respected Catholic high schools. At the strip shopping center to your right on Robert E. Lee, you have a few options for coffee and a snack: Tutti Frutti Frozen Yogurt; Chateau Café; and PJ's Coffee, inside Robért Fresh Market.

POINTS OF INTEREST

Brisbi's brisbisrestaurant.com, 7400 Lakeshore Drive, 504-304-4125

The Blue Crab thebluecrabnola.com, 7900 Lakeshore Drive, 504-284-2898

Landry's Seafood landrysseafood.com, 8000 Lakeshore Drive, 504-283-1010

New Canal Lighthouse Museum and Education Center saveourlake.org, 8001 Lakeshore Drive, 504-282-2134

Tutti Frutti Frozen Yogurt tfyogurt.com, 143 Robert E. Blvd., 504-304-8530

Chateau Café chateaucafe.com, 139 Robert E. Lee Blvd., 504-286-1777

PJ's Coffee at Robért Fresh Market pjscoffee.com/node/180, 153 Robert E. Lee Blvd., 504-282-3100

route summary

1. Begin walk at Robert E. Lee Boulevard and Lakeshore Drive.

2. Facing Lakeshore, turn right (north) and walk about 0.75 mile to Lake Pontchartrain.

3. Circle right on Lakeshore Drive and walk about a mile to Marconi Drive.

4. Turn right on Marconi, walk eight blocks to Robert E. Lee, and turn right.

5. Walk 14 blocks back to the starting point.

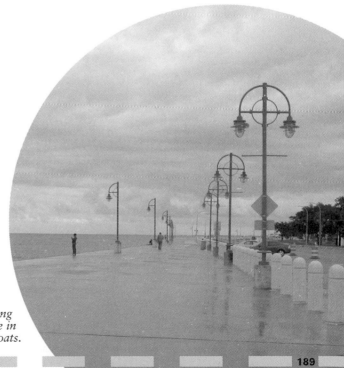

*Lakeshore Drive, which runs along
Lake Pontchartrain, is the perfect place to take in
a sunset and view passing boats.*

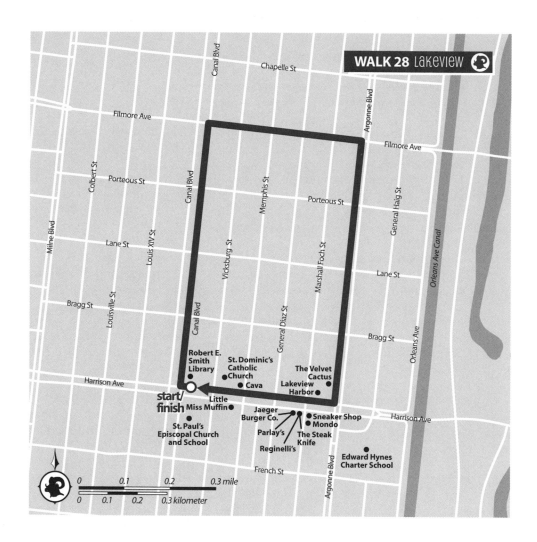

WALK 28 Lakeview

Chapelle St

Canal Blvd

Argonne Blvd

Filmore Ave

Filmore Ave

Colbert St

Porteous St

Memphis St

Porteous St

General Haig St

Milne Blvd

Lane St

Louis XIV St

Canal Blvd

Vicksburg St

Marshall Foch St

Orleans Ave Canal

Lane St

Bragg St

Louisville St

Canal Blvd

General Diaz St

Bragg St

Orleans Ave

Robert E.
Smith
Library

St. Dominic's
Catholic
Church

The Velvet
Cactus

Harrison Ave

Cava

Lakeview
Harbor

**start/
finish**

Little
Miss Muffin

Jaeger
Burger Co.

Sneaker Shop

Mondo

Harrison Ave

St. Paul's
Episcopal Church
and School

Parlay's

The Steak
Knife

Reginelli's

Edward Hynes
Charter School

Argonne Blvd

French St

0   0.1   0.2   0.3 mile

0   0.1   0.2   0.3 kilometer

28 Lakeview: From Debris to Delight

BOUNDARIES: Canal Blvd., Filmore Ave., Argonne Blvd., Harrison Ave.
DISTANCE: 1.56 miles
PARKING: Free on the street and the Harrison Ave. neutral ground
PUBLIC TRANSIT: RTA Bus #45 (Lakeview)

Imagine your neighborhood wiped out by a powerful hurricane, its winds ripping off roofs and water from a nearby levee breach reaching as high as 9 feet.

Residents of Lakeview didn't have to imagine it—they lived it. On August 29, 2005, Hurricane Katrina obliterated this upper-middle-class community, destroying its homes along with its quality of life. Many residents drowned, unable or unwilling to evacuate in the days leading up to the storm.

While many survivors relocated to other parts of the country or to less-affected parts of New Orleans, others vowed to rebuild. Improvements in levee strength and flood control helped their cause, and today the neighborhood is as strong and vibrant as ever.

Lakeview is considered one of the safest areas of New Orleans, and most residents have no qualms about taking an evening stroll to Harrison Avenue, where they can shop at Lakeview Grocery, grab dinner at chef Susan Spicer's Mondo, or splurge on an ice-cream cone at The Creole Creamery.

Activities abound in Lakeview as well, from church and school fairs to the monthly Harrison Avenue Marketplace, sponsored by the Friends of Lakeview and the Lakeview Civic Improvement Association. The event features an art market, music, and food from area restaurants.

● Begin in front of Robert E. Smith Library, one of 14 branches of the New Orleans Public Library. Like the rest of Lakeview, the old library was flooded so badly that it had to be rebuilt from the ground up. The process took more than six years, but when the new building finally opened in 2012, it was bigger and better than ever. In addition to 40,000 volumes, the 12,700-square-foot library has a colorful, fully stocked children's corner, 17 computers, meeting space, and a self-checkout system.

- Turn right on Canal Boulevard and walk four blocks to Filmore Avenue. Canal Boulevard, which runs from City Park Avenue to Lake Pontchartrain, is actually an extension of Canal Street, which runs from City Park Avenue to the Mississippi River. Canal Boulevard is largely a residential thoroughfare divided by a parklike neutral ground. Due to the breach of the 17th Street Canal—on the west side of Lakeview—no one escaped the Katrina flooding in this neighborhood. Consequently, houses were either restored or, like the library, built anew. It's easy to spot the new ones: Many are two- and three-story mansions, some of which dwarf their neighbors. Others are restored early-20th-century cottages and bungalows. Almost all of the houses were built high off the ground.

- Turn right on Filmore and walk five blocks to Argonne Boulevard. As you walk, imagine the piles of debris that littered the neighborhood during the Katrina recovery process. Many residents lived in trailers provided by the Federal Emergency Management Agency (FEMA), and for a long time, Lakeview resembled a mammoth mobile-home park.

- Turn right on Argonne Boulevard and walk four blocks to Harrison Avenue. Before Katrina, Argonne was one of the most attractive streets in Lakeview, and it is once again, with most homes sporting lush and meticulously maintained gardens and lawns.

- Turn right onto Harrison, Lakeview's main commercial strip. At the corner is The Velvet Cactus, one of several new restaurants that have opened in Lakeview since Katrina. The Mexican restaurant's relaxing patio is great for sipping a pineapple-cilantro margarita or any number of other tropical drinks. Inside, the walls are adorned with the works of local artists, and most of the art is for sale.

As you make the turn on Harrison, take note of the building across the street and to your left: That's Edward Hynes Charter School, long one of the city's top-rated public schools. After Katrina, the original school building was torn down to make way for this new state-of-the art-campus. Students, at least those who returned to New Orleans, were schooled in temporary quarters while construction ensued. When the new Hynes opened in January 2012—more than six years after the storm—it was considered a crucial step in the neighborhood's recovery.

- As you continue down Harrison, you'll pass an assortment of businesses, from salons to banks. Some, like Jaeger Burger Co. and Cava (a bar and bistro), are new to Lakeview since Katrina, while others, like the Sneaker Shop (a shoe store) and Lakeview Harbor (a burger joint), are longtime fixtures. One of the most celebrated newcomers is Mondo, chef Susan Spicer's "flavors of the world" eatery. In opening Mondo in 2010, Spicer, a Lakeview resident, felt strongly about bringing a new dining concept to the neighborhood. She succeeded, with crowds flocking to the eatery daily for dishes like Thai shrimp-and-pork meatballs, Szechuan eggplant stir-fry, and wood-fired pizzas.

- Walk one block. To the left is a strip of businesses that include The Steak Knife, a neighborhood steakhouse; Reginelli's, part of a local pizza chain; and Parlay's, a legendary corner bar that claims to have the longest bar in New Orleans, at 60 feet.

- Walk one block to Memphis Street. To the right is St. Dominic's Catholic Church, one of the largest in New Orleans. St. Dominic's parish dates back to 1924, though Lakeview's first formal place of Catholic worship—a small wooden chapel on nearby Chapelle Street—opened in 1912. As Lakeview grew, so did St. Dominic's need for a larger worship space, and in 1961 it moved to its current location on Harrison. Behind it is St. Dominic's Catholic School, which serves students in pre-kindergarten through grade 7. One of the most memorable days in the church's history occurred on November 27, 2005, when St. Dominic's held its first Mass three months after Katrina. The church had been gutted, and there was still no electricity or residents in Lakeview. But that didn't matter to church parishioners who came from far and wide to attend the service. "This is the nucleus that holds this community together, and this is the nucleus that's going to bring the community back," a parishioner told USA Today.

Across Harrison from Smith Library is St. Paul's Episcopal Church and School, which got its start in a small room at Lee Circle in downtown New Orleans in the 1830s. Like St. Dominic's, St. Paul's moved several times before settling into its current digs on Canal Boulevard. It struggled to survive after Katrina, as illustrated on its website: "For three weeks the church and school sat under eight feet of polluted water and debris. The result was the total destruction of the first-floor interiors as well as two single-story buildings that had to be demolished. With 80 percent of the city flooded and businesses ruined, the tragic scattering of our people ensued." With the help of volunteers from around the country, St. Paul's plunged into the rebuilding process, transforming mountains of debris into a source of pride. But it didn't just help itself—it helped all of Lakeview, opening a Homecoming Center to help restore lives and rebuild homes. Today, its services include raising money for communities that have experienced similar disasters.

● Your walk ends at this corner. If you want a quick bite to eat or a sip of something cold, check out Nola Beans, at 762 Harrison, or The Creole Creamery, around the corner at 6260 Vicksburg St. And be sure to stop at Little Miss Muffin (766 Harrison), a whimsical boutique next door to Nola Beans that sells everything from children's clothing to home-decor items.

POINTS OF INTEREST

Robert E. Smith Library tinyurl.com/robertesmithlibrary, 6301 Canal Blvd., 504-596-2638

The Velvet Cactus thevelvetcactus.com, 6300 Argonne Blvd., 504-301-2083

Lakeview Harbor 911 Harrison Ave., 504-486-4887

Sneaker Shop 904 Harrison Ave., 504-488-9919

Mondo mondoneworleans.com, 900 Harrison Ave., 504-224-2633

The Steak Knife thesteakkniferestaurant.com, 888 Harrison Ave., 504-488-8981

Reginelli's Pizzeria reginellis.com, 874 Harrison Ave., 504-488-0133

Jaeger Burger Co. jaegerburger.homestead.com, 872 Harrison Ave., 504-482-1441

Parlay's parlaysbar.net, 870 Harrison Ave., 504-304-6338

Cava tinyurl.com/cavanola, 789 Harrison Ave., 504-304-9034

Little Miss Muffin shoplittlemissmuffin.com, 766 Harrison Ave., 504-482-8200

Nola Beans nolabeans.com, 762 Harrison Ave., 504-267-0783

The Creole Creamery creolecreamery.com, 6260 Vicksburg St., 504-482-2924

route summary

1. Begin walk at corner of Canal Boulevard and Harrison Avenue.
2. Walk four blocks to Filmore Avenue and turn right.
3. Walk five blocks to Argonne Boulevard and turn right.
4. Walk four blocks back to Harrison and turn right.
5. Walk five blocks back to starting point.

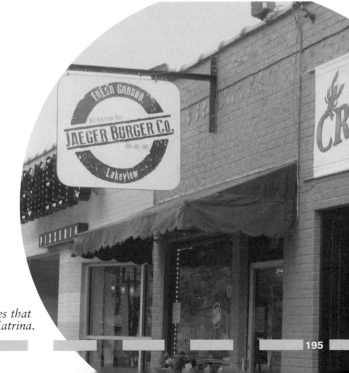

Jaeger Burger Co. is one of several new eateries that have sprung up in Lakeview since Hurricane Katrina.

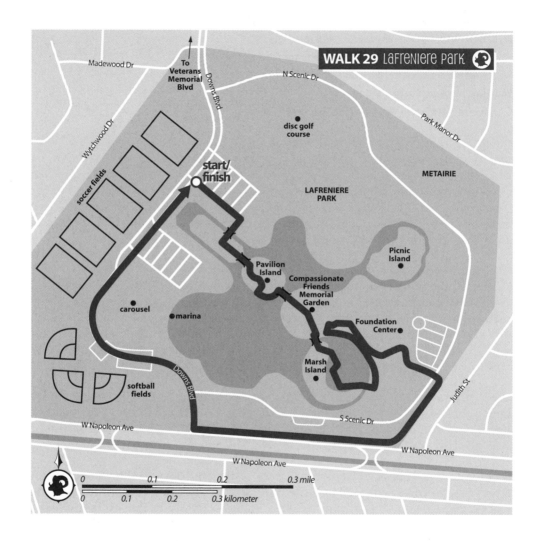

Madewood Dr

To
Veterans
Memorial
Blvd

N Scenic Dr

Downs Blvd

Park Manor Dr

Wytchwood Dr

soccer fields

disc golf
course

METAIRIE

start/
finish

LAFRENIERE
PARK

Picnic
Island

Pavilion
Island

Compassionate
Friends
Memorial
Garden

carousel

marina

Foundation
Center

Marsh
Island

softball
fields

Downs Blvd

Judith St

S Scenic Dr

W Napoleon Ave

W Napoleon Ave

W Napoleon Ave

0   0.1   0.2   0.3 mile
0   0.1   0.2   0.3 kilometer

29 Lafreniere Park: Suburban Sanctuary

BOUNDARIES: **David Dr., Wytchwood Dr., Madewood Dr., Park Manor Dr., Judith St.,**
W. Napoleon Ave.
DISTANCE: **1.5 miles**
PARKING: **Free parking throughout park**
PUBLIC TRANSIT: **Jefferson Transit Bus E1 (Veterans)**

Big-box stores, chain restaurants, and strip shopping centers—they pretty much define
Veterans Memorial Boulevard in Metairie, a sprawling suburb just west of New Orleans.
But thanks to the efforts of a citizens' group back in the early 1970s, the 155-acre Lafreniere
Park was born, becoming the center of recreational life in what would become one of the
most populous areas of southern Louisiana. Named after Nicolas Chauvin de la Frénière,
a former Louisiana attorney general who inherited the land in the mid-18th century, the park
opened in 1982, after voters approved a bond issue to acquire the land.

Over the past three decades, the park has evolved into a destination, inviting tourists and
locals alike to take in its fountains, lagoons, gardens, and trails. Among the park's highlights is a boardwalk through Marsh Island, a wildlife habitat where visitors can easily
spot such species as ibis, sandpipers, geese, swans, and egret. For children, the park offers
a 4,000-square-foot spray park and an old-fashioned carousel. If they play soccer, chances
are they'll be competing at Lafreniere, which has five soccer fields and four softball fields.
The park's newest additions are Bark Park (a gated dog park) and a disc golf course.

Lafreniere is home to some of the area's most popular holiday events, including the Uncle
Sam Jam, a Fourth of July extravaganza; Park-a-Boo, a Halloween shindig for children; and
Holiday in the Park, a spectacular Christmas-light display with a 60-foot sea serpent in the
lagoon, a princess and her magical castle, and the gingerbread man.

● **From Veterans Memorial Boulevard, drive south on Downs Boulevard, cross over**
North Scenic Drive, and pull into the parking lot to the left. Start off by walking south-
west along Downs across from the park's soccer fields. To the left is the first of
many lakes that you'll see as you make your way around the park. Benches surround
the lake, making it a pleasant spot to read a book or pose for photos.

- Walk past the lake and turn left. Continue walking and cross the first bridge. This will take you to the concert pavilion, where many festivals take place. Turn south at the pavilion toward the lake, where ducks and other waterfowl make their home. Circle around until you see another bridge. This one leads to a circular garden, where markers tell the history of the park. This is also the location of the Compassionate Friends Memorial Garden. Each year, Compassionate Friends, a nonprofit support group for parents and families who have lost a child, holds a memorial walk in the park.

- Continue walking south until you reach the park's boardwalk bridge, which winds through Marsh Island, a natural wildlife habitat. Listen for the sounds of crickets, ducks, and the occasional crowing rooster. Squirrels, turtles, rabbits, raccoons, nutria, and opossums also call the island home. In the middle of the boardwalk is a small pavilion where you can stop and marvel at the sight of geese, swans, and ducks floating in the lake.

- As you step off the boardwalk, don't be surprised to encounter ducks, ibis, and other wildlife hanging out on the pathways and the shores of the lake. Continue circling until you see a trash receptor to the right. Turn right, walk a few feet to the jogging trail, and take another right on the trail. On the left are the park's administrative offices and the Foundation Room, the park's special-events venue.

- Cross South Scenic Drive and continue on the jogging trail. Be wary of joggers, who tend to pack the park on weekends. As you stroll on the trail, you'll see a warm-up station where visitors can stretch before running. As the trail winds through the back of the park, you'll see a picnic pavilion to the right and baseball fields to the left.

- Cross South Scenic Drive and walk toward another lake. Turn left at the path and continue walking around the lake. If it's summertime, you'll soon hear the sounds of children frolicking in the spray park. On the other side is a carousel, which, unlike the spray park, is open all year. A nearby snack bar offers a variety of cool treats, though hours vary.

- Walk toward Downs and turn right before crossing the street. Walk past the soccer fields and cross over several parking lots until you reach the lot where you started.

POINTS OF INTEREST

Lafreniere Park lafrenierepark.org, 3000 Downs Blvd., Metairie; 504-838-4389

route summary

1. Enter park from intersection of Veterans and Downs Boulevards.
2. Park in lot on left and head south along Downs.
3. Turn left at corner of Downs and walk to bridge.
4. Cross over series of bridges.
5. Walk across boardwalk through Marsh Island.
6. Turn right at first trash receptor and get on jogging trail.
7. Follow trail around park until you reach Downs.
8. Turn right on Downs and walk to starting point.

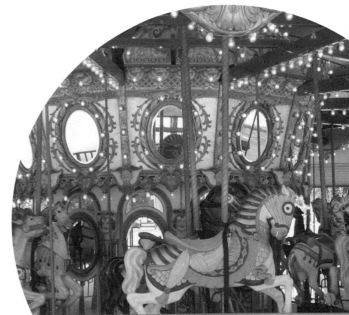

The carousel at Lafreniere Park boasts 30 moving horses, a tiger, a zebra, and two chariots.

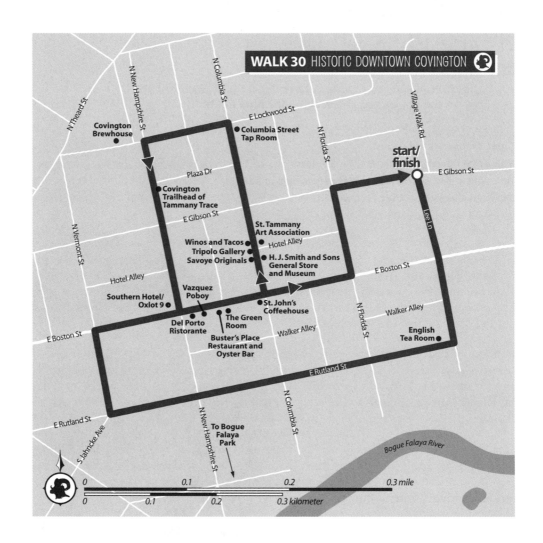

WALK 30 HISTORIC DOWNTOWN COVINGTON

N Theard St
N New Hampshire St
N Columbia St
E Lockwood St
Village Walk Rd

Covington Brewhouse
Columbia Street Tap Room

N Florida St

Plaza Dr

start/ finish
E Gibson St

Covington Trailhead of Tammany Trace

Lee Ln

E Gibson St

N Vernont St

St. Tammany Art Association

Winos and Tacos
Hotel Alley
Tripolo Gallery
Savoye Originals
H. J. Smith and Sons General Store and Museum

E Boston St

Hotel Alley

Vazquez Poboy
Southern Hotel/ Oxlot 9
St. John's Coffeehouse

Del Porto Ristorante
The Green Room
Walker Alley
N Florida St
Walker Alley

Buster's Place Restaurant and Oyster Bar
English Tea Room

E Boston St
E Rutland St

E Rutland St

S Jahncke Ave
N New Hampshire St
To Bogue Falaya Park
N Columbia St

Bogue Falaya River

0   0.1   0.2   0.3 mile

0   0.1   0.2   0.3 kilometer

30 HISTORIC DOWNTOWN COVINGTON: a STEP BACK IN TIME

BOUNDARIES: E. Rutland St., Lee Lane, E. Lockwood St., N. Vermont St.
PARKING: Free on the street, but check signs for time limits.
DISTANCE: 1.38 miles
PUBLIC TRANSIT: None

St. Tammany Parish, on the North Shore of Lake Pontchartrain, is home to a thriving collection of communities, from Abita Springs to Madisonville to Slidell. The city of Covington is among them, boasting such attractions as riverside parks, horse farms, and a historic downtown district.

Founded as the town of Wharton in 1813 but later renamed after Gen. Leonard Covington, a War of 1812 hero, the so-called Three Rivers community lies at the fork of the Bogue Falaya, Tchefuncte, and Abita Rivers. The downtown area thrived for decades but fell victim to the oil bust of 1986, forcing many businesses to shut down. In 1987, the city applied to and was accepted into the National Main Street Program, a downtown-revitalization initiative that started Covington's comeback in 1992.

The downtown district combines historic landmarks such as the Southern Hotel and H. J. Smith & Son General Store and Museum with modern and hip destinations such as Winos and Tacos, St. John's Coffeehouse, and the Green Room. Unique to the city is its grid layout, featuring squares-within-squares, or ox lots, that are accessible through alleyways and are now used for public parking.

The area also boasts a performing-arts center, a microbrewery, and several bed-and-breakfasts, all just steps away from the Bogue Falaya River and Bogue Falaya Park. Numerous art galleries also dot the streets, and every year, the Three River Arts Festival enhances the area's reputation as an arts and art lovers' Mecca.

● **Begin on Lee Lane and East Gibson Street. Facing Lee Lane, turn left and walk two blocks to East Rutland Street. Lee Lane is a quaint two-block stretch of boutiques,** galleries, and restaurants. These include Ballin's, a high-end clothing store; Walker House Collectibles, housed in a classic Southern cottage; and Bella Cucina, which sells pestos, oils, spices, and other Italian ingredients.

- Turn right on East Rutland and walk four blocks to North Vermont Street. On this part of the walk, you'll pass many turn-of-the-century cottages, some of which have been converted to businesses such as the English Tea Room at 734 East Rutland. East Rutland also has several bed-and-breakfasts, including Blue Willow and Camellia House. At the intersection of East Rutland and North Columbia Street, to the left, is the Columbia Street Landing, which sits along the banks of the Bogue Falaya River. Bogue Falaya Park is just off North New Hampshire Street. The park is not included on this tour, but feel free to detour and then make your way back to East Rutland.

- At North Vermont Street, turn right and then right again onto East Boston Street, the district's main drag. At 428 E. Boston is the newly renovated Southern Hotel, which opened in 1907 as a retreat for visitors who enjoyed the nearby piney woods and mineral springs. The hotel closed in the 1960s, and over the next several decades, the property housed a drugstore, government offices, and courthouses. After Hurricane Katrina, it served as the headquarters for the Red Cross and various federal agencies. Local developers bought the property in 2011 and set out to restore and reopen it as a luxury hotel. In addition to its 42 guest rooms, the hotel has a lush courtyard, a ballroom, an upscale bar, a fitness room, and spa services. Its restaurant, Oxlot 9, boasts an award-winning chef, Jeffrey Hansell, who has worked with the likes of chefs Tory McPhail (Commander's Palace) and John Besh (Domenica, Borgne, Restaurant August, etc.). Other dining destinations on East Boston include Del Porto Ristorante, Buster's Place Restaurant and Oyster Bar, and Vazquez Poboy.

- Walk two blocks to North Columbia Street, cross East Boston, and walk three blocks to East Lockwood Street. North Columbia is an art lover's haven, with numerous galleries, cafés, specialty shops, and antiques stores lining the street. They include Tripolo Gallery, which represents more than a dozen artists, and Savoye Originals, known for functional art made of recycled and reclaimed materials. Stop in H. J. Smith and Sons General Store and Museum, a Covington institution since 1876. The store sells everything from hardware and army surplus to coonskin caps and rubber boots. Among the items on display at the museum are a hand-operated washing machine, a 1920s gas pump, and other memorabilia from the 1870s through the early part of the 20th century.

- Just down the block at 320 N. Columbia is the home of the St. Tammany Art Association, which was founded in 1958 by a small group of individuals dedicated to bringing the arts to west St. Tammany Parish. The association helps promote emerging and established artists, in addition to offering arts education and exhibitions. Every year, the group sponsors the Geaux Arts Ball, which raises money for its educational-outreach program.

  Across the street at 321 N. Columbia is Winos and Tacos, a fun spot to chill with a glass of wine or a margarita. The Columbia Street Tap Room, at 434 N. Columbia, serves 30 beers on tap and 60 varieties of bottled beer.

- Turn left at East Lockwood Street and walk one block to North New Hampshire Street. At this intersection you'll see the Covington Brewhouse, where craft beers such as Pontchartrain Pilsner, Bayou Bock, and Kölsch are microbrewed. The brewery is open for tours on Saturdays from 10 a.m. to noon.

- Turn left on North New Hampshire and stop at the Covington Trailhead, which marks the beginning of a 31-mile paved trail called the Tammany Trace. The trail connects Covington with the cities of Abita Springs, Mandeville, Lacombe, and Slidell. The site has a clock tower, an amphitheater, a museum and visitor center, and a small movie theater. You'll also see the world's tallest statue of President Ronald Reagan. On Wednesdays, the Covington Farmers Market sets up shop here, selling locally grown fruits and vegetables as well as locally produced eggs, milk, cheese, meat, poultry, and seafood. Musical performances and cooking demonstrations add to the festivities.

- Walk two blocks back to East Boston Street, then turn left and walk two blocks to North Florida Street. If you need a place to rest your feet and sip a drink, The Green Room music club (521 E. Boston) begins its happy hour at 2 p.m. For lattes and other coffee drinks, try St. John's Coffeehouse, at 535 E. Boston.

- At North Florida, turn left and walk one block to East Gibson Street. Turn right and walk one block back to the starting point on Lee Lane.

POINTS OF INTEREST

English Tea Room englishtearoom.com, 734 E. Rutland St., Covington; 985-898-3988

Bogue Falaya Park tinyurl.com/boguefalayapark, 213 Park Drive, Covington; 985-892-1873

Southern Hotel southernhotel.com, 428 E. Boston St., Covington; 985-871-5223

Oxlot 9 oxlot9.com, 428 E. Boston St., Covington; 985-400-5663

Del Porto Ristorante delportoristorante.com, 501 E. Boston St., Covington; 985-875-1006

Vazquez Poboy vazquezpoboy.com, 515 E. Boston St., Covington; 985-893-9336

Buster's Place Restaurant and Oyster Bar bustersplaceonline.com, 519 E. Boston St., Covington; 985-809-3880

H. J. Smith and Sons General Store and Museum 308 N. Columbia St., Covington; 985-892-0460

St. Tammany Art Association sttammanyartassociation.org, 320 N. Columbia St., Covington; 985-892-8650

Tripolo Gallery tripologallery.com, 323 N. Columbia St., Covington; 985-789-4073

Winos and Tacos 321 N. Columbia St., Covington; 985-809-3029

Savoye Originals Gallery tinyurl.com/savoyeoriginals, 405 N. Columbia St., Covington; 504-512-3465

Columbia Street Tap Room covingtontaproom.com, 434 N. Columbia St., Covington; 985-898-0899

Covington Brewhouse covingtonbrewhouse.com, 226 E. Lockwood St., Covington; 888-910-2337

Tammany Trace, Covington Trailhead tammanytrace.org, 419 N. New Hampshire St., Covington; 866-892-1873

The Green Room greenroomcovla.com, 521 E. Boston St., Covington; 985-892-2225

St. John's Coffeehouse stjohnscoffeehouse.com, 535 E. Boston St., Covington; 985-893-5553

rouTe summary

1.   Begin walk on Lee Lane.
2.   Walk two blocks to East Rutland Street and turn right.
3.   Walk four blocks to North Vermont Street and turn right.
4.   Walk one block to East Boston Street and turn right.
5.   Walk two blocks to North Columbia Street and cross East Boston, heading north.
6.   Walk three blocks to East Lockwood Street and turn left.
7.   Walk one block to North New Hampshire Street and turn left.
8.   Walk two blocks to East Boston and turn left.
9.   Walk two blocks to North Florida Street and turn left.
10. Walk one block to East Gibson Street and turn right.

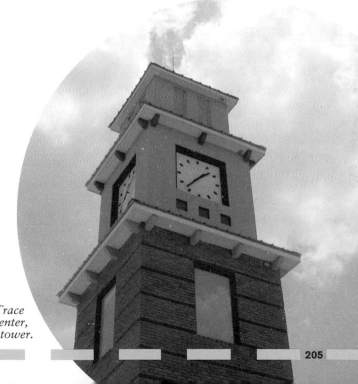

The Covington Trailhead of the Tammany Trace
features a bandstand, a visitor center,
and this clock tower.

Appendix 1: WALKS BY THEME

GREEN SPACES

Audubon Park (Walk 13)

Bogue Falaya Park (Walk 30, Historic Downtown Covington)

Chalmette Battlefield and National Cemetery (Walk 24)

City Park (Walk 18)

Coliseum Square (Walk 7, Lower Garden District)

Crescent Park (Walk 22, Bywater)

Jackson Square (Walk 4, French Quarter)

Jean Lafitte Barataria Preserve (Walk 26)

Lafayette Square (Walk 1, Warehouse District)

Lafreniere Park (Walk 29)

Lakeshore Drive (Walk 27, Lakefront)

Louis Armstrong Park (Walk 20, Treme)

Washington Square (Walk 21, Faubourg Marigny)

Woldenberg Riverfront Park (Walk 6, Riverfront/French Market)

WATER, WATER EVERYWHERE

Bayou St. John (Walk 19, Faubourg St. John)

Big Lake (Walk 18, City Park)

Lake Pontchartrain (Walk 27, Lakefront)

Louisiana wetlands (Walk 26, Jean Lafitte Barataria Preserve)

Mississippi River (Walk 6, Riverfront/French Market; Walk 13, Audubon Park; Walk 22, Bywater; Walk 25, Algiers Point)

DINING, SHOPPING, AND ENTERTAINMENT

Bywater (Walk 22)

Esplanade Avenue (Walk 19, Faubourg St. John)

French Quarter (Walk 4, French Quarter; Walk 5, Back of the Quarter; Walk 6, Riverfront/French Market)

Frenchmen Street (Walk 21, Faubourg Marigny)

Freret Street (Walk 14)

Harrah's New Orleans (Walk 2, Canal Street; Walk 3, Poydras Street)

Harrison Avenue (Walk 28, Lakeview)

Lee Lane (Walk 30, Historic Downtown Covington)

Magazine Street (Walk 11)

North Carrollton Avenue (Walk 17, Mid-City)

Oak Street (Walk 16, Carrollton)

Riverbend (Walk 16, Carrollton)

The Shops at Canal Place (Walk 2, Canal Street)

Warehouse District (Walk 1)

MUSEUMS

Backstreet Cultural Museum
(Walk 20, Treme)
The Cabildo (Walk 4, French Quarter)
Chalmette Battlefield Visitor Center
(Walk 24)
Confederate Memorial Hall Museum
(Walk 1, Warehouse District)
Contemporary Arts Center
(Walk 1, Warehouse District)
**H. J. Smith and Sons General Store and
Museum** (Walk 30, Historic Downtown
Covington)
Historic New Orleans Collection
(Walk 4, French Quarter)
Louisiana Children's Museum
(Walk 1, Warehouse District)
Lower Ninth Ward Living Museum
(Walk 23, Lower Ninth Ward)
National World War II Museum
(Walk 1, Warehouse District)
**New Orleans African American Museum of
Art, Culture and History**
(Walk 20, Treme)
**New Canal Lighthouse Museum and
Education Center** (Walk 27, Lakefront)
New Orleans Museum of Art
(Walk 18, City Park)
Ogden Museum of Southern Art
(Walk 1, Warehouse District)
Old US Mint (Walk 5, Back of the Quarter;
Walk 21, Faubourg Marigny)
Pharmacy Museum (Walk 4, French Quarter)
Pitot House (Walk 19, Faubourg St. John)

Southern Food and Beverage Museum
(Walk 8, Oretha Castle Haley Boulevard)
The Presbytère (Walk 4, French Quarter)

ART, INSIDE AND OUT

Audubon Park (Walk 13)
Contemporary Arts Center (Walk 1,
Warehouse District)
Julia Street (Walk 1, Warehouse District)
Louis Armstrong Park (Walk 20, Treme)
Magazine Street (Walk 11)
New Orleans Museum of Art
(Walk 18, City Park)
North Columbia Street
(Walk 30, Historic Downtown Covington)
Ogden Museum of Southern Art
(Walk 1, Warehouse District)
Royal Street (Walk 4, French Quarter)
**Sydney and Walda Besthoff Sculpture
Garden** (Walk 18, City Park)
Woldenberg Riverfront Park (Walk 6,
Riverfront/French Quarter)

FAMILY FUN

Audubon Aquarium of the Americas
(Walk 6, Riverfront/French Quarter)
Audubon Butterfly Garden and Insectarium
(Walk 2, Canal Street)
Audubon Park and Audubon Zoo (Walk 13)
Canal Street (Walk 2)
City Park (Walk 18)

Appendix 2: POINTS OF INTEREST

CEMETERIES

Canal Street Cemeteries (Cities of the Dead) saveourcemeteries.org (Walk 17)

Lafayette No. 1 Cemetery saveourcemeteries.org/lafayette-cemetery-no-1, 1400 Washington Ave., 504-658-3781 (Walk 10)

St. Louis Cemetery No. 1 saveourcemeteries.org, 320 N. Claiborne Ave., 504-596-3050 (Walk 20)

St. Louis Cemetery No. 3 saveourcemeteries.org, 3421 Esplanade Ave., 504-482-5065 (Walk 19)

MUSIC MANIA

Apple Barrel tinyurl.com/applebarrelnola, 609 Frenchmen St., 504-949-9399 (Walk 21)

Blue Nile bluenilelive.com, 532 Frenchmen St., 504-948-2583 (Walk 21)

Balcony Music Club 1331 Decatur St., 504-522-2940 (Walk 21)

Café Negril 606 Frenchmen St., 504-944-4744 (Walk 21)

Candlelight Lounge 925 N. Robertson St., 504-525-4748 (Walk 20)

d.b.a. dbaneworleans.com, 618 Frenchmen St., 504-942-3731 (Walk 21)

Famous Door 339 Bourbon St., 504-598-4334 (Walk 4)

Freret Street Publiq House publiqhouse.com, 4528 Freret St., 504-826-9912 (Walk 14)

Gasa Gasa gasagasa.com, 4920 Freret St., Twitter: @gasagasanola (Walk 14)

The Green Room greenroomcovla.com, 521 E. Boston St., Covington; 985-892-2225 (Walk 30)

Igor's Checkpoint Charlie's 501 Esplanade Ave., 504-281-4847 (Walk 21)

Irvin Mayfield's Jazz Playhouse irvinmayfield.com, 300 Bourbon St., 504-553-2299 (Walk 4)

Le Bon Temps Roulé 4801 Magazine St., 504-895-8117 (Walk 11)

Little Gem Saloon littlegemsaloon.com, 445 S. Rampart St., 504-267-4863 (Walk 3)

Louisiana Music Factory louisianamusicfactory.com, 421 Frenchmen St., 504-586-1094 (Walk 21)

The Maison maisonfrenchmen.com, 508 Frenchmen St., 504-371-5543 (Walk 21)

Maple Leaf Bar mapleleafbar.com, 8316 Oak St., 504-866-9359 (Walk 16)

Miss Jean's Famous Corner Courtyard tinyurl.com/missjeans, 437 Esplanade Ave., 504-252-4800 (Walk 21)

Old Point Bar 545 Patterson Drive, 504-364-0950 (Walk 25)

Palm Court Jazz Cafe palmcourtjazzcafe.com, 1204 Decatur St., 525-0200 (Walk 6)

Preservation Hall preservationhall.com, 726 St. Peter St., 504-522-2841 (Walk 4)

Snug Harbor snugjazz.com, 626 Frenchmen St., 504-949-0696 (Walk 21)

Spotted Cat spottedcatmusicclub.com, 623 Frenchmen St. (no phone) (Walk 21)

Vaso facebook.com/vasonola, 500 Frenchmen St., 504-272-0929 (Walk 21)

Something Sweet

Adrian's Bakery adrians-bakery.com, 2016 Oretha Castle Haley Blvd., 504-875-4302 (Walk 8)

Angelo Brocato's angelobrocatoicecream.com/aboutus.shtm, 214 N. Carrollton Ave., 504-486-1465 (Walk 17)

Beaucoup Juice facebook.com/beaucoupjuice, 4719 Freret St., 504-430-5508 (Walk 14)

Blue Dot Donuts bluedotdonuts.com, 4301 Canal St., 504-218-4866 (Walk 17)

Blue Frog Chocolates bluefrogchocolates.com, 5707 Magazine St., 504-269-5707 (Walk 11)

Café Du Monde cafedumonde.com, 800 Decatur St., 504-525-4544 (Walk 6)

CC's Coffee House ccscoffeehouse.com, 900 Jefferson Ave., 504-891-4969 (Walk 11); 2800 Esplanade Ave., 504-482-9865 (Walk 19)

Chateau Café chateaucafe.com, 139 Robert E. Lee Blvd., 504-286-1777 (Walk 27)

Church Alley Coffee Bar churchalleycoffeebar.tumblr.com, 1618 Oretha Castle Haley Blvd.,
Twitter: @churchalley (Walk 8)

The Creole Creamery creolecreamery.com, 6260 Vicksburg St., 504-482-2924 (Walk 28)

District: Donuts Sliders Brew donutsandsliders.com, 2209 Magazine St., 504-570-6945
(Walk 9)

EnVie Espresso Bar & Cafe nolalovescoffee.com/envie-espresso-bar-cafe, 1241 Decatur St.,
504-524-3689 (Walk 6)

Kupcakes Etc. kupcakesetc.angelfire.com, 501 Pelican Ave., 504-364-9384 (Walk 25)

Mojo Coffee House facebook.com/mojofreret, 4700 Freret St., 504-875-2243 (Walk 14)

Morning Call neworleanscitypark.com/in-the-park/morning-call, 56 Dreyfous Drive,
504-300-1157 (Walk 18)

Nola Beans nolabeans.com, 762 Harrison Ave., 504-267-0783 (Walk 28)

Piety Street Sno-Balls 612 Piety St., 504-782-2569 (Walk 22)

PJ's Coffee at Stern Hall pjscoffee.com, 7001 Freret St., 504-865-5705 (Walk 15)

PJ's Coffee at Robért Fresh Market pjscoffee.com/node/180, 153 Robert E. Lee Blvd.,
504-282-3100 (Walk 27)

Pure Cake purecakenola.com, 5035 Freret St., 504-872-0065 (Walk 14)

Rue de la Course facebook.com/ruedelacourse, 1140 S. Carrollton Ave., 504-861-4343
(Walk 16)

St. John's Coffeehouse stjohnscoffeehouse.com, 535 E. Boston St., Covington;
985-893-5553 (Walk 30)

Still Perkin' neworleanscoffeeshop.com, 2727 Prytania St., 504-899-0335 (Walk 10)

Sucré shopsucre.com, 3025 Magazine St., 504-520-8311 (Walk 9)

The Rook Café facebook.com/therookcafe, 4516 Freret St., 618-520-9843 (Walk 14)

Tutti Frutti Frozen Yogurt tfyogurt.com, 143 Robert E. Blvd., 504-304-8530 (Walk 27)

Village Coffee and Tea villagecoffeenola.com, 5335 Freret St., 504-861-1909 (Walk 14)

FOOD AND DRINK

Acme Oyster House acmeoyster.com, 724 Iberville St., 504-522-5973 (Walk 4)

Adolfo's tinyurl.com/adolfosnola, 611 Frenchmen St., 504-948-3800 (Walk 21)

Ancora Pizzeria & Salumeria ancorapizza.com, 4508 Freret, 504-324-1636 (Walk 14)

Apolline apollinerestaurant.com, 4729 Magazine St., 504-894-8869 (Walk 11)

Audubon Clubhouse Café auduboninstitute.org/visit/clubhouse-cafe, 6500 Magazine St., 504-212-5282 (Walk 13)

Avo (opens spring 2015) 5908 Magazine St. (Walk 11)

Bamboula's bamboulasnola.com, 514 Frenchmen St., 504-944-8461 (Walk 21)

Bar Tonique bartonique.com, 820 N. Rampart St., 504-324-6045 (Walk 20)

Bistro Daisy bistrodaisy.com, 5831 Magazine St., 504-899-6987 (Walk 11)

The Blue Crab thebluecrabnola.com, 7900 Lakeshore Drive, 504-284-2898 (Walk 27)

Booty's Street Food bootysnola.com, 800 Louisa St., 504-266-2887 (Walk 22)

Borgne borgnerestaurant.com, 601 Loyola Ave., 504-613-3860 (Walk 3)

Bourbon House bourbonhouse.com, 144 Bourbon St., 504-522-0111 (Walk 4)

Brisbi's brisbisrestaurant.com, 7400 Lakeshore Drive, 504-304-4125 (Walk 27)

Brown Butter Southern Kitchen & Bar brownbutterrestaurant.com, 231 N. Carrollton Ave., 504-609-3871 (Walk 17)

Bud's Broiler budsbroiler.com, 500 City Park Ave., 504-486-2559 (Walk 17)

The Bulldog bulldog.draftfreak.com, 3236 Magazine St., 504-891-1516 (Walk 9)

Buster's Place Restaurant and Oyster Bar bustersplaceonline.com, 519 E. Boston St., Covington; 985-809-3880 (Walk 30)

Café Adelaide cafeadelaide.com, 300 Poydras St., 504-595-3305 (Walk 3)

Café Amelie cafeamelie.com, 912 Royal St., 504-412-8965 (Walk 5)

Café Degas cafedegas.com, 3127 Esplanade Ave., 504-945-5635 (Walk 19)

Café Minh cafeminh.com, 4139 Canal St., 504-482-6266 (Walk 17)

Café Reconcile cafereconcile.org, 1631 Oretha Castle Haley Blvd., 504-568-1157 (Walk 8)

Café Rose Nicaud caferosenicaud.com, 632 Frenchmen St., 504-949-3300 (Walk 21)

Cajun Brothers Seafood & Poboys facebook.com/cajunbrothersseafood, 236 N. Carrollton Ave., 504-488-7503 (Walk 17)

Camellia Grill 626 S. Carrollton Ave., 504-309-2679 (Walk 16)

Cane & Table caneandtablenola.com, 1113 Decatur St., 504-581-1112 (Walk 6)

Carousel Bar & Lounge, Hotel Monteleone hotelmonteleone.com, 214 Royal St., 504-523-3341 (Walk 4)

Carrollton Market carrolltonmarket.com, 8132 Hampson St., 504-252-9928 (Walk 16)

Casa Borrega casaborrega.com, 1719 Oretha Castle Haley Blvd., 504-427-0654 (Walk 8)

Casamento's casamentosrestaurant.com, 4330 Magazine St., 504-895-9761 (Walk 11)

Cava tinyurl.com/cavanola, 789 Harrison Ave., 504-304-9034 (Walk 28)

Central Grocery 923 Decatur St., 504-523-1620 (Walk 6)

Chiba chiba-nola.com, 8312 Oak St., 504-826-9119 (Walk 16)

Chris Owens Club chrisowensclub.net, 500 Bourbon St., 504-523-6400 (Walk 4)

Columbia Street Tap Room covingtontaproom.com, 434 N. Columbia St., Covington; 985-898-0899 (Walk 30)

The Columns Hotel thecolumns.com, 3811 St. Charles Ave., 504-899-9308 (Walk 12)

Commander's Palace commanderspalace.com, 1403 Washington Ave., 504-899-8221 (Walk 10)

The Company Burger thecompanyburger.com, 4600 Freret St., 504-267-0320 (Walk 14)

Coop's Place coopsplace.net, 1109 Decatur St., 504-525-9053 (Walk 6)

Cooter Brown's cooterbrowns.com, 509 S. Carrollton Ave., 504-866-9104 (Walk 16)

Coquette coquettenola.com, 2800 Magazine St., 504-265-0421 (Walk 9)

The Country Club thecountryclubneworleans.com, 634 Louisa St., 504-945-0742 (Walk 22)

Crêpes à la Cart crepecaterer.com, 1039 Broadway St., 504-866-2362 (Walk 15)

Crown & Anchor English Pub crownanchorpub.com, 200 Pelican Ave., 504-227-1007 (Walk 25)

Cure curenola.com, 4905 Freret St., 504-302-2357 (Walk 14)

Dat Dog datdognola.com, 3336 Magazine St., 504-324-2226 (Walk 9); 5030 Freret St., 504-899-6883 (Walk 14); 601 Frenchmen St., 504-309-3362 (Walk 21)

The Delachaise thedelachaise.com, 3442 St. Charles Ave., 504-895-0858 (Walk 12)

Del Porto Ristorante delportoristorante.com, 501 E. Boston St., Covington; 985-875-1006 (Walk 30)

Dickie Brennan's Steakhouse dickiebrennanssteakhouse.com, 716 Iberville St., 504-522-2467 (Walk 4)

Domenica domenicarestaurant.com, 123 Baronne St., 504-648-6020 (Walk 2)

Doris Metropolitan dorismetropolitan.com, 620 Chartres St., 504-267-3500 (Walk 4)

Drago's Seafood Restaurant dragosrestaurant.com, 2 Poydras St., 504-584-3911 (Walk 3)

Dry Dock Café thedrydockcafe.com, 133 Delaronde St., 504-361-8240 (Walk 25)

Emeril's emerilsrestaurants.com, 800 Tchoupitoulas St., 504-528-9393 (Walk 1)

English Tea Room englishtearoom.com, 734 E. Rutland St., Covington; 985-898-3988 (Walk 30)

Fat Harry's fatharrysneworleans.com, 4330 St. Charles Ave., 504-895-9582 (Walk 12)

Felix's Restaurant and Oyster Bar felixs.com, 739 Iberville St., 504-522-4440 (Walk 4)

Frady's One Stop Food Store 3231 Dauphine St., 504-949-9688 (Walk 22)

French Market frenchmarket.org, 1235 N. Peters St., 504-596-3420 (Walk 6)

Freret Street Po-Boy and Donut Shop freretstreetpoboys.com, 4701 Freret St., 504-872-9676 (Walk 14)

Fulton Alley fultonalley.com, 600 Fulton St., 504-208-5569 (Walk 3)

Galatoire's galatoires.com, 209 Bourbon St., 504-525-2021 (Walk 4)

Garden District Pub gardendistrictpub.com, 1916 Magazine St., 504-267-3392 (Walk 7)

Golden Feather Mardi Gras Indian Restaurant Gallery goldenfeatherneworleans.com, 704 N. Rampart St., 504-266-2339 (Walk 20)

Good Friends Bar goodfriendsbar.com, 740 Dauphine St., 504-566-7191 (Walk 5)

Grand Isle Restaurant grandislerestaurant.com, 575 Convention Center Blvd., 504-520-8540 (Walk 3)

Happy's Irish Pub happysirishpub.com, 1009 Poydras St., 504-304-9236 (Walk 3)

Harrah's New Orleans harrahsneworleans.com, 228 Poydras St., 800-427-7247 (Walks 2 and 3)

Harry's Corner 900 Chartres St., 504-524-1107 (Walk 5)

Henry's Uptown Bar facebook.com/henrys.uptown.bar, 5101 Magazine St., 504-324-8140 (Walk 11)

High Hat Café highhatcafe.com, 4500 Freret St., 504-754-1336 (Walk 14)

Hillel's Kitchen hknola.com, 912 Broadway St., 504-909-9919 (Walk 15)

Humble Bagel humblebagel.com, 4716 Freret St., 504-355-3535 (Walk 14)

Irene's Cuisine 539 St. Philip St., 504-529-8811 (Walk 5)

Ivy ivynola.com, 5015 Magazine St., 504-899-1330 (Walk 11)

Jacques-Imo's jacques-imos.com, 8324 Oak St., 504-861-0886 (Walk 16)

Jaeger Burger Co. jaegerburger.homestead.com, 872 Harrison Ave., 504-482-1441 (Walk 28)

Jean Lafitte's Old Absinthe House ruebourbon.com/oldabsinthehouse, 240 Bourbon St., 504-523-3181 (Walk 4)

Jimmy Buffett's Margaritaville margaritavilleneworleans.com, 1104 Decatur St., 504-592-2565 (Walk 6)

Johnny Sánchez New Orleans johnnysanchezrestaurant.com, 930 Poydras St., 504-304-6615 (Walk 3)

Juan's Flying Burrito juansflyingburrito.com, 2018 Magazine St., 504-569-0000 (Walk 7)

Juicy Lucy's msjuicylucy.com, 133 N. Carrollton Ave., 504-598-5044 (Walk 17)

K-Paul's Louisiana Kitchen chefpaul.com/kpaul, 416 Chartres St., 504-596-2530 (Walk 4)

Kingfish cocktailbarneworleans.com, 337 Chartres St., 504-598-5005 (Walk 4)

Lafitte's Blacksmith Shop lafittesblacksmithshop.com, 941 Bourbon St., 504-593-9761 (Walk 5)

Lakeview Harbor 911 Harrison Ave., 504-486-4887 (Walk 28)

Landry's Seafood landrysseafood.com, 8000 Lakeshore Drive, 504-283-1010 (Walk 27)

La Petite Grocery lapetitegrocery.com, 4238 Magazine St., 504-891-3377 (Walk 11)

Liberty Cheesesteaks libertycheesesteaks.com, 5031 Freret St., 504-875-4447 (Walk 14)

Lilette liletterestaurant.com, 3637 Magazine St., 504-895-1636 (Walk 11)

Liuzza's by the Track liuzzasnola.com, 1518 N. Lopez St., 504-218-7888 (Walk 19)

Lola's lolasneworleanscom, 3312 Esplanade Ave., 504-488-6946 (Walk 19)

Madigan's Bar 800 S. Carrollton Ave., 504-866-9455 (Walk 16)

Manning's harrahsneworleans.com/restaurants.html, 519 Fulton St., 504-593-8118 (Walk 1)

Marigny Brasserie marignybrasserie.com, 640 Frenchmen St., 504-945-4472 (Walk 21)

Markey's Bar facebook.com/markeysbarnola, 640 Louisa St., 504-943-0785 (Walk 22)

Maurepas Foods maurepasfoods.com, 3200 Burgundy St., 504-267-0072 (Walk 22)

Mayas mojitoland.com, 2027 Magazine St., 504-309-3401 (Walk 7)

Meauxbar meauxbar.com, 942 N. Rampart St., 504-569-9979 (Walk 20)

Midway Pizza midwaypizzanola.com, 4725 Freret St., 504-322-2815 (Walk 14)

The Milk Bar 710 S. Carrollton Ave., 504-309-3310 (Walk 12)

Mint Modern Bistro & Bar mintmodernbistro.com, 5100 Freret St., 504-218-5534 (Walk 14)

Mondo mondoneworleans.com, 900 Harrison Ave., 504-224-2633 (Walk 28)

Molly's at the Market mollysatthemarket.net, 1107 Decatur St., 504-525-5169 (Walk 6)

Mother's Restaurant mothersrestaurant.net, 401 Poydras St., 504-523-9656 (Walk 3)

MoPho mophonola.com, 514 City Park Ave., 504-482-6845 (Walk 17)

Ms. Mae's msmaeswallofshame.blogspot.com, 4336 Magazine St., 504-218-8035 (Walk 11)

Mulate's mulates.com, 201 Julia St., 504-522-1492 (Walk 1)

Muriel's Jackson Square muriels.com, 801 Chartres St., 504-568-1885 (Walk 4)

Napoleon House napoleonhouse.com, 500 Chartres St., 504-524-9752 (Walk 4)

New Orleans Hamburger & Seafood Company nohsc.com, 4141 St. Charles Ave., 504-247-9753 (Walk 12)

Nonna Mia nonnamia.net, 3125 Esplanade Ave., 504-948-1717 (Walk 19)

Oak Wine Bar oaknola.com, 8118 Oak St., 504-302-1485 (Walk 16)

O'Henry's Food & Spirits ohenrys.com, 632 Carrollton Ave., 504-866-9741 (Walk 16)

Origami Sushi sushinola.com, 5130 Freret St., 504-899-6532 (Walk 14)

Oxalis oxalisbywater.com, 3162 Dauphine St., 504-267-4776 (Walk 22)

Oxlot 9 oxlot9.com, 428 E. Boston St., Covington; 985-400-5663 (Walk 30)

Palace Café palacecafe.com, 605 Canal St., 504-523-1661 (Walk 2)

Parasol's parasolsbarandrestaurant.com, 2533 Constance St., 504-302-1543 (Walk 9)

Parlay's parlaysbar.net, 870 Harrison Ave., 504-304-6338 (Walk 28)

Pat O'Brien's patobriens.com, 718 St. Peter St., 504-525-4823 (Walk 4)

Pêche Seafood Grill pecherestaurant.com, 800 Magazine St., 504-522-1744

Pho Bistreaux phobistreaux.biz, 1200 S. Carrollton Ave., 504-304-8334 (Walk 16)

Pizza Delicious pizzadelicious.com, 617 Piety St., 504-676-8482 (Walk 22)

Pizza Domenica pizzadomenica.com, 4933 Magazine St., 504-301-4978 (Walk 11)

Port of Call portofcallnola.com, 838 Esplanade Ave., 504-523-0120 (Walks 5 and 21)

The Praline Connection pralineconnection.com, 542 Frenchmen St., 504-943-3934 (Walk 21)

Purloo nolapurloo.com, 1504 Oretha Castle Haley Blvd., 504-324-6020 (Walk 8)

R Bar royalstreetinn.com/r-bar, 1431 Royal St., 504-948-7499 (Walk 21)

Ralph's On the Park ralphsonthepark.com, 900 City Park Ave., 504-488-1000 (Walk 18)

Refuel Café refuelcafe.com, 8124 Hampson St., 504-872-0187 (Walk 16)

Reginelli's Pizzeria reginellis.com, 5961 Magazine St., 504-899-1414 (Walk 11); 874 Harrison Ave., 504-488-0133 (Walk 28)

Reservoir Café reservoircafe.com, 2045 Magazine St., 504-324-5633 (Walk 7)

Restaurant R'evolution revolutionnola.com, 777 Bienville St., 504-553-2277 (Walk 4)

Root rootnola.com, 200 Julia St., 504-252-9480 (Walk 1)

Rue 127 rue127.com, 127 N. Carrollton Ave., 504-483-1571 (Walk 17)

Roux Carré (opens 2015) goodworknetwork.org/foodcourt, 2000 Oretha Castle Haley Blvd., 504-309-2073

The Rum House Caribbean Taqueria rumhousenola.com, 3128 Magazine St., 504-941-7560 (Walk 9)

Ruth's Chris Steak House ruthschris.com, 525 Fulton St., 504-587-7099 (Walk 3)

Saints and Sinners saintsandsinnersnola.com, 627 Bourbon St., 504-528-9307 (Walk 4)

Sake Café Uptown sakecafeuptown.us, 2830 Magazine St., 504-894-0033 (Walk 9)

Salu salurestaurant.com, 3226 Magazine St., 504-371-5809 (Walk 9)

Santa Fe santafenola.com, 3201 Esplanade Ave., 504-948-0077 (Walk 19)

Sarita's Grill 4520 Freret St., 504-324-3562 (Walk 14)

Satsuma Cafe satsumacafe.com, 3218 Dauphine St., 504-304-5962 (Walk 22)

Saturn Bar saturnbar.com, 3067 St. Claude Ave., 504-949-7532 (Walk 22)

Slim Goodies Diner slimgoodiesdiner.com, 3322 Magazine St., 504-891-3447 (Walk 9)

SoBou sobounola.com, 310 Chartres St., 504-552-4095 (Walk 4)

Square Root squarerootnola.com, 1800 Magazine St., 504-309-7800 (Walk 7)

Stanley stanleyrestaurant.com, 547 St. Ann St., 504-587-0093 (Walk 4)

The Steak Knife thesteakkniferestaurant.com, 888 Harrison Ave., 504-488-8981 (Walk 28)

Stein's Market & Deli steinsdeli.net, 2207 Magazine St., 504-527-0771 (Walk 9)

Sugar Park sugarparknola.com, 3054 St. Claude Ave., 504-942-2047 (Walk 22)

Superior Seafood superiorseafoodnola.com, 4338 St. Charles Ave., 504-293-3474 (Walk 12)

Superior Grill superiorgrill.com, 3636 St. Charles Ave., 504-899-4200 (Walk 12)

Surrey's Uptown surreycafeandjuicebar.com, 4807 Magazine St., 504-895-5757 (Walk 11)

Sylvain sylvainnola.com, 625 Chartres St., 504-265-8123 (Walk 4)

Tableau tableaufrenchquarter.com, 616 St. Peter St., 504-934-3463 (Walk 4)

13 Monaghan Bar 13monaghan.com, 517 Frenchmen St., 504-942-1345 (Walk 21)

Three Muses 3musesnola.com, 536 Frenchmen St., 504-252-4801 (Walk 21)

Tout de Suite Cafe toutdesuitecafe.com, 347 Verret St., 504-362-2264 (Walk 25)

Tracey's traceysnola.com, 2604 Magazine St., 504-897-5413 (Walk 9)

Tropical Isle tropicalisle.com, 600 Bourbon St., 504-529-1702 (Walk 4)

Truburger truburgernola.com, 8115 Oak St., 504-218-5416 (Walk 16)

Tujague's Restaurant tujaguesrestaurant.com, 823 Decatur St., 504-525-8676 (Walk 6)

Vazquez Poboy vazquezpoboy.com, 515 E. Boston St., Covington; 985-893-9336 (Walk 30)

The Velvet Cactus thevelvetcactus.com, 6300 Argonne Blvd., 504-301-2083 (Walk 28)

Venezia venezianeworleans.net, 134 N. Carrollton Ave., 504-488-7991 (Walk 17)

Verti Marte 1201 Royal St., 504-525-4767 (Walk 5)

Vine & Dine vine-dine.com, 141 Delaronde St., 504-361-1402 (Walk 25)

Walk-On's Bistreaux & Bar walk-ons.com, 1009 Poydras St., 504-309-6530 (Walk 3)

Wayfare wayfarenola.com, 4510 Freret St., 504-309-4510 (Walk 14)

Whole Foods Market–Arabella Station wholefoodsmarket.com/stores/arabellastation, 5600 Magazine St., 504-899-9119 (Walk 11)

Winos and Tacos 321 N. Columbia St., Covington; 985-809-3029 (Walk 30)

Wit's Inn witsinn.com, 141 N. Carrollton Ave., 504-486-1600 (Walk 17)

educational and cultural centers

Ashé Cultural Arts Center ashecac.org, 1712 Oretha Castle Haley Blvd., 504-569-9070 (Walk 8)

Audubon Aquarium of the Americas auduboninstitute.org/visit/aquarium, 1 Canal St., 504-565-3033 (Walk 6)

Audubon Insectarium auduboninstitute.org/visit/insectarium, 423 Canal St., 504-524-2847 (Walk 2)

Basin St. Station basinststation.com, 501 Basin St., 504-293-2600 (Walk 20)

Cabrini High School cabrinihigh.com, 1400 Moss St., 504-482-1193 (Walk 19)

Covington Brewhouse covingtonbrewhouse.com, 226 E. Lockwood St., Covington; 888-910-2337 (Walk 30)

Entergy IMAX Theatre auduboninstitute.org/visit/imax, 1 Canal St., 504-565-3033 (Walk 6)

House of Broel houseofbroel.com, 2220 St. Charles Ave., 504-522-2220 (Walk 10)

Indywood Cinema indywood.org, 628 Elysian Fields Ave., 504-345-8804 (Walk 21)

International School of Louisiana isl-edu.org, 1400 Camp St., 504-654-1088 (Walk 7)

Jazz Walk of Fame nps.gov/jazz, Algiers–Canal Street Ferry Terminal, 504-589-4841 (Walk 25)

Jewish Community Center nojcc.org, 5342 St. Charles Ave., 504-897-0143

Joy Theater thejoytheater.com, 1200 Canal St., 504-528-9569 (Walk 2)

La Nuit Comedy Theater nolacomedy.com, 5039 Freret St., 504-231-7011

Le Petit Théâtre du Vieux Carré lepetittheatre.com, 616 St. Peter St., 504-522-2081 (Walk 4)

Loyola University New Orleans loyno.edu, 6363 St. Charles Ave., 504-865-3240 (Walk 15)

Mercedes-Benz Superdome superdome.com, 1500 Sugar Bowl Drive, 504-587-3663 (Walk 3)

New Orleans Jazz Market 1436 Oretha Castle Haley Blvd. (still under construction as of this writing) (Walk 8)

New Orleans Jazz National Historical Park nps.gov/jazz, 916 N. Peters St., 504-589-4841 (Walk 6)

New Orleans Women's Opera Guild Home operaguildhome.org, 2504 Prytania St., 504-899-1945 (Walk 10)

Robert E. Smith Library tinyurl.com/robertesmithlibrary, 6301 Canal Blvd., 504-596-2638 (Walk 28)

Saenger Theatre saengernola.com, 1111 Canal St., 504-525-1052 (Walk 2)

St. Alphonsus Art and Cultural Center stalphonsusneworleans.org, 2025 Constance St., 504-524-8116 (Walk 9)

Tulane University tulane.edu, 6823 St. Charles Ave., 504-865-5000 (Walk 15)

Zeitgeist Multi-Disciplinary Arts Center zeitgeistinc.net, 1618 Oretha Castle Haley Blvd., 504-827-5858 (Walk 8)

MUSEUMS

African American Museum of Art, Culture and History noaam.org, 1418 Governor Nicholls St., 504-566-1136 (Walk 20)

Backstreet Cultural Museum backstreetmuseum.org 1116 Henriette Delille St., 504-522-4806 (Walk 20)

Beauregard-Keyes House bkhouse.org, 1113 Chartres St., 504-523-7257 (Walk 5)

The Cabildo crt.state.la.us/louisiana-state-museum, 701 Chartres St., 504-568-6968 (Walk 4)

Confederate Memorial Hall Museum confederatemuseum.com, 922 Camp St., 504-523-4522 (Walk 1)

Contemporary Arts Center cacno.org, 900 Camp St., 504-528-3805 (Walk 1)

Historic New Orleans Collection hnoc.org, 522 Royal St., 504-523-4662 (Walk 4)

H. J. Smith and Sons General Store and Museum 308 N. Columbia St., Covington; 985-892-0460 (Walk 30)

Louisiana Children's Museum lcm.org, 420 Julia St., 504-523-1357 (Walk 1)

Lower Ninth Ward Living Museum l9livingmuseum.org, 1235 Deslonde St., 504-220-3652 (Walk 23)

National World War II Museum nationalww2museum.org, 945 Magazine St., 504-527-6012 (Walk 1)

New Canal Lighthouse Museum and Education Center saveourlake.org, 8001 Lakeshore Drive, 504-282-2134 (Walk 27)

New Orleans Museum of Art noma.org, 1 Collins Diboll Circle, 504-658-4100 (Walk 18)

Ogden Museum of Southern Art ogdenmuseum.org, 925 Camp St., 504-539-9650 (Walk 1)

Old US Mint crt.state.la.us, 400 Esplanade Ave., 504-568-2022 (Walks 5 and 21)

Pharmacy Museum pharmacymuseum.org, 514 Chartres St., 504-565-8027 (Walk 4)

Pitot House louisianalandmarks.org, 1440 Moss St., 504-482-0312 (Walk 19)

The Presbytère crt.state.la.us/louisiana-state-museum, 751 Chartres St., 504-568-6968 (Walk 4)

Southern Food and Beverage (SoFAB) Culinary Library and Archive sofabinstitute.org /sofab-culinary-library-and-archive, 1609 Oretha Castle Haley Blvd., 504-569-0405 (Walk 8)

Southern Food and Beverage Museum (SoFAB) sofabinstitute.org, 1504 Oretha Castle Haley Blvd., 504-569-0405 (Walk 8)

Tammany Trace, Covington Trailhead tammanytrace.org, 419 N. New Hampshire St., Covington; 866-892-1873 (Walk 30)

outdoor recreation and parks

Audubon Park and Audubon Zoo auduboninstitute.org, 6500 Magazine St., 504-581-4629 (Walk 13)

Audubon Golf Course auduboninstitute.org/visit/golf, 6500 Magazine St., 504-861-2537 (Walk 13)

Barataria Preserve, Jean Lafitte National Historical Park nps.gov/jela/barataria-preserve .htm, 6588 Barataria Blvd., Marrero; 504-689-3690, Ext. 10 (Walk 26)

Bogue Falaya Park tinyurl.com/boguefalayapark, 213 Park Drive, Covington; 985-892-1873 (Walk 30)

Cabrini Playground Dauphine Street between Governor Nicholls and Barracks Streets (Walk 5)

Carousel Gardens Amusement Park neworleanscitypark.com/in-the-park/carousel-gardens, Victory Avenue, 504-483-9402 (Walk 18)

City Park neworleanscitypark.com, 1 Palm Drive, 504-428-4888 (Walks 17, 18, and 19)

City Putt neworleanscitypark.com/in-the-park/city-putt, 8 Victory Ave., 504-483-9385 (Walk 18)

Coliseum Square Park 1700 Coliseum St. (Walk 7)

Confetti Park 451 Pelican Ave. at Verret Street (Walk 25)

Crescent Park reinventingthecrescent.org, Mississippi River between Elysian Fields Avenue and Mazant Street, 504-658-4334 (Walk 22)

Danneel Playspot 5501 St. Charles Ave. at Octavia Street (Walk 12)

Desmare Playground 3456 Esplanade Ave. between Esplanade and Moss Street (Walk 19)

The Fly auduboninstitute.org/audubon-park/favorites/the-riverview, 504-861-2537 (Walk 13)

Fortier Park Bounded by Esplanade Avenue, Grand Route St. John, and Mystery Street (Walk 19)

Friday Night Fights Gym 1630 Oretha Castle Haley Blvd., 504-522-2707 (Walk 8)

Jackson Square nola.gov/parks-and-parkways/parks-squares/jackson-square, St. Ann, St. Peter, Decatur, and Chartres Streets; 504-658-3200 (Walk 4)

Lafayette Square nola.gov/parks-and-parkways/parks-squares/lafayette-square, bounded by St. Charles Ave., Camp St., N. Maestri St., and S. Maestri St.; 504-658-3200 (Walk 1)

Lafitte Greenway (opens spring 2015) Basin Street to Canal Boulevard, folc-nola.org, 504-462-0645 (Walk 17)

Lafreniere Park lafrenierepark.org, 3000 Downs Blvd., Metairie; 504-838-4389 (Walk 29)

Louis Armstrong Park nola.gov/parks-and-parkways/parks-squares/congo-square -louis-armstrong-park, 701 N. Rampart St., 504-658-3200 (Walk 20)

McDonogh Park Bounded by Bermuda, Verret, and Alix Streets (Walk 25)

Mickey Markey Park 700 Piety St. (Walk 22)

New Orleans Botanical Garden neworleanscitypark.com/botanical-garden, 3 Victory Ave., 504-483-4888 (Walk 18)

Steamboat *Natchez* steamboatnatchez.com, Toulouse Street Wharf, 504-569-1401 (Walk 6)

Storyland neworleanscitypark.com/in-the-park/storyland, 7 Victory Ave., 504-483-4888 (Walk 18)

Tammany Trace, Covington Trailhead tammanytrace.org, 419 N. New Hampshire St., Covington; 866-892-1873 (Walk 30)

Woldenberg Riverfront Park auduboninstitute.org/visit/aquarium/exhibits-and-attractions /woldenberg-park, 1 Canal St., 504-565-3033 (Walk 6)

Historic Landmarks

Academy of the Sacred Heart ashrosary.org, 4521 St. Charles Ave., 504-891-1943 (Walk 12)

Algiers Courthouse friendsofalgierscourthouse.org, 225 Morgan St. (Walk 25)

Blessed Francis Xavier Seelos Catholic Church seeloschurchno.org, 3053 Dauphine St., 504-943-5566 (Walk 22)

Chalmette Battlefield and National Cemetery nps.gov/jela/chalmette-battlefield.htm, 8606 W. St. Bernard Highway, Chalmette; 504-281-0510 (Walk 24)

Cita Dennis Hubbell Library hubbelllibrary.org, 725 Pelican Ave., 504-596-3113 (Walk 25)

Cornstalk Hotel cornstalkhotel.com, 915 Royal St., 504-523-1515 (Walk 5)

Gallier House hgghh.org, 1132 Royal St., 504-525-5661 (Walk 5)

Holy Name of Jesus Church hnjchurch.org, 6367 St. Charles Ave., 504-865-7430 (Walk 15)

House of the Rising Sun Bed and Breakfast risingsunbnb.com, 335 Pelican Ave., 504-231-6498 (Walk 25)

Hurricane Katrina Memorial North Claiborne Avenue between Tennessee and Reynes Streets (Walk 23)

John Minor Wisdom US Court of Appeals Building tinyurl.com/jmwbuilding, 600 Camp St., 504-310-7700 (Walk 1)

LaLaurie House 1140 Royal St. (Walk 5)

Milton H. Latter Memorial Library tinyurl.com/nolapubliclibraries, 5120 St. Charles Ave., 504-596-2625 (Walk 12)

Louise S. McGehee School mcgeheeschool.com, 2343 Prytania St., 504-561-1224 (Walk 10)

Louisiana Supreme Court lasc.org, 400 Royal St., 504-310-2300 (Walk 4)

Madame John's Legacy crt.state.la.us/louisiana-state-museum, 632 Dumaine St., 504-568-6968 (Walk 5)

Miltenberger Houses 900, 906, and 910 Royal St. (Walk 5)

Mortuary Haunted House hauntedmortuary.com, 4800 Canal St., 504-483-2350 (Walk 17)

Mount Olivet Episcopal Church mountolivet.org, 530 Pelican Ave., 504-366-4650 (Walk 25)

New Orleans Police Department, Eighth District nola.gov/nopd, 334 Royal St., 504-658-6080

New Orleans Women's Opera Guild Home operaguildhome.org, 2504 Prytania St., 504-899-1945 (Walk 10)

Old St. Patrick's Church oldstpatricks.org, 724 Camp St., 504-525-4413 (Walk 1)

Old Ursuline Convent oldursulineconvent.org, 1100 Chartres St., 504-529-3040 (Walk 5)

Our Lady of the Rosary Catholic Church ourladyoftherosary-no.com, 3368 Esplanade Ave., 504-488-2659 (Walk 19)

Robert E. Lee Monument St. Charles Ave. at Lee Circle (Walk 1)

Roosevelt Hotel therooseveltneworleans, 130 Roosevelt Way, 504-648-1200 (Walk 2)

Soniat House soniathouse.com, 1133 Chartres St., 504-522-0570 (Walk 5)

Southern Hotel southernhotel.com, 428 E. Boston St., Covington; 985-871-5223 (Walk 30)

St. Augustine Catholic Church staugustinecatholicchurch-neworleans.org, 1210 Governor Nicholls St., 504-525-5934 (Walk 20)

St. Alphonsus Art and Cultural Center stalphonsusneworleans.org, 2025 Constance St., 504-524-8116 (Walk 9)

St. Louis Cathedral stlouiscathedral.org, Jackson Square, 504-525-9585 (Walk 4)

St. Vincent's Guest House stvguesthouse.com, 1507 Magazine St., 504-302-9606 (Walk 7)

Touro Synagogue tourosynagogue.com, 4238 St. Charles Ave., 504-895-4843 (Walk 12)

Trinity Lutheran Church sites.google.com/site/trinityalgierspoint, 620 Eliza St., 504-368-0411 (Walk 25)

Washington Artillery Park frenchmarket.org/venue/washington-artillery-park, 749 Decatur St., 504-596-3420 (Walk 6)

Galleries and Public Art

Audubon Park auduboninstitute.org, 6500 Magazine St., 504-581-4629 (Walk 13)

Arthur Roger Gallery arthurrogergallery.com, 432 Julia St., 504-522-1999 (Walk 1)

Carol Robinson Gallery carolrobinsongallery.com, 840 Napoleon Ave., 504-895-6130 (Walk 11)

Dutch Alley Artist's Co-op dutchalleyartistsco-op.com, 912 N. Peters St., 504-412-9220 (Walk 6)

Frenchy Gallery frenchylive.com, 8319 Oak St., 504-861-7595 (Walk 16)

Jean Bragg Gallery jeanbragg.com, 600 Julia St., 504-895-7375 (Walk 1)

Jonathan Ferrara Gallery jonathanferraragallery.com, 400-A Julia St., 504-522-5471 (Walk 1)

LeMieux Galleries lemieuxgalleries.com, 332 Julia St., 504-522-5988 (Walk 1)

Martine Chaisson Gallery martinechaissongallery.com, 727 Camp St., 504-302-7942 (Walk 1)

Michalopoulos Studio michalopoulos.com, 527 Elysian Fields Ave., 504-558-0505 (Walk 21)

Newcomb Art Gallery newcombartgallery.tulane.edu, Newcomb Quad, 504-865-5328 (Walk 15)

OCH Art Market ochartmarket.com, 1618 Oretha Castle Haley Blvd., 985-250-0278 (Walk 8)

Rosetree Blown Glass Studio rosetreegallery.com, 446 Vallette St., 888-767-8733 (Walk 25)

Søren Christensen sorengallery.com, 400 Julia St., 504-569-9501 (Walk 1)

Savoye Originals Gallery tinyurl.com/savoyeoriginals, 405 N. Columbia St., Covington; 504-512-3465 (Walk 30)

St. Tammany Art Association sttammanyartassociation.org, 320 N. Columbia St., Covington; 985-892-8650 (Walk 30)

Sydney and Walda Besthoff Sculpture Garden noma.org, 1 Collins Diboll Circle, 504-658-4100 (Walk 18)

Thomas Mann Gallery I/O thomasmann.com, 1812 Magazine St., 504-581-2113 (Walk 7)

Tripolo Gallery tripologallery.com, 323 N. Columbia St., Covington; 985-789-4073 (Walk 30)

Woldenberg Riverfront Park auduboninstitute.org/visit/aquarium/exhibits-and-attractions/woldenberg-park, 1 Canal St., 504-565-3033 (Walk 6)

SHOPPING

Adler's adlersjewelry.com, 722 Canal St., 504-523-5292 (Walk 2)

Aidan Gill for Men aidangillformen, 2026 Magazine St., 504-587-9090 (Walk 7)

Algiers Music Point algiersmusicpoint.com, 323 Verret St., 504-304-4201 (Walk 25)

American Aquatic Gardens americanaquaticgardens.com, 621 Elysian Fields Ave., 504-944-0410 (Walk 21)

The Bank Architectural Antiques thebankantiques.com, 1824 Felicity St., 504-523-2702 (Walk 8)

Bargain Center 3200 Dauphine St., 504-948-0007 (Walk 22)

Bead Shop beadshopneworleans.com, 4612 Magazine St., 504-895-6161 (Walk 11)

Bootsy's Funrock'n facebook.com/funrockn.popcity, 3109 Magazine St., 504-895-4102 (Walk 9)

Brad and Dellwen Flag Party 2201 Magazine St., 504-527-5211 (Walk 9)

Campus Connection campusconnection.cc, 800 Broadway St., 504-866-8552 (Walk 15)

Charlie Boy facebook.com/charlieboynola, 2043 Oretha Castle Haley Blvd., Instagram: @charlieboynola (Walk 8)

Dirty Coast dirtycoast.com, 5631 Magazine St., 504-324-3745 (Walk 11)

EarthSavers earthsaversonline.com, 5501 Magazine St., 504-899-8555 (Walk 11)

Eclectic Home eclectichome.net, 8211 Oak St., 504-866-6654 (Walk 16)

Euclid Records www.euclidnola.com, 3301 Chartres St., 504-947-4348 (Walk 22)

Fleurty Girl fleurtygirl.net, 3117 Magazine St., 504-301-2557 (Walk 9)

Funky Monkey funkymonkeynola.com, 3127 Magazine St., 504-899-5587 (Walk 9)

Garden District Book Shop gardendistrictbookshop.com, 2727 Prytania St., 504-895-2266 (Walk 10)

Glue Clothing Exchange glueclothingexchange.com, 8206 Oak St., 504-782-0619 (Walk 16)

Green Serene greenserenenola.com, 2041 Magazine St., 504-252-9861 (Walk 7)

Haase's haases.com, 8119 Oak St., 504-866-9944 (Walk 16)

Hazelnut hazelnutneworleans.com, 5515 Magazine St., 504-891-2424 (Walk 11)

H. J. Smith and Sons General Store and Museum 308 N. Columbia St., Covington; 985-892-0460 (Walk 30)

I. J. Reilly's Knick-Knacks and Curiosities ijreillys.squarespace.com, 632 Elysian Fields Ave., 504-304-7928 (Walk 21)

Jax Brewery jacksonbrewery.com, 600 Decatur St., 504-566-7245 (Walk 6)

Judy at the Rink facebook.com/judyattherink, 2727 Prytania St., 504-891-7018 (Walk 10)

Little Miss Muffin shoplittlemissmuffin.com, 766 Harrison Ave., 504-482-8200 (Walk 28)

Marie Laveau's House of Voodoo voodooneworleans.com, 739 Bourbon St., 504-581-3751 (Walk 5)

Mid-City Market mid-citymarket.com, 401 N. Carrollton Ave. (Walk 17)

Miette iheartmiette.com, 2038 Magazine St., 504-522-2883 (Walk 7)

Mignon mignonnola.com, 2727 Prytania St., 504-891-2374 (Walk 10)

Mignon Faget mignonfaget.com, 3801 Magazine St., 504-891-2005 (Walk 11)

Mimi miminola.com, 5500 Magazine St., 504-269-6464 (Walk 11)

The Mushroom facebook.com/mushroomnola, 1037 Broadway St., 504-866-6065 (Walk 15)

NOLA Couture nolacouture.com, 2928 Magazine St., 504-319-5959 (Walk 9)

Outlet Collection at Riverwalk riverwalkneworleans.com, 500 Port of New Orleans, 504-522-1555 (Walk 1)

Pippen Lane pippenlane.com, 2930 Magazine St., 504-269-0106 (Walk 9)

Pop Shop 3212 Dauphine St. (no phone or website) (Walk 22)

Rubensteins rubensteinsneworleans.com, 102 St. Charles Ave., 504-581-6666 (Walk 2)

The Shops at Canal Place theshopsatcanalplace.com, 333 Canal St., 504-522-9200 (Walk 2)

Sneaker Shop 904 Harrison Ave., 504-488-9919 (Walk 28)

Spring springboutique.net, 5525 Magazine St., 504-896-9185 (Walk 11)

Trashy Diva trashydiva.com, 2048 Magazine St., 504-299-8777 (Walk 7)

Tubby & Coo's Mid-City Book Shop tubbyandcoos.com, 631 N. Carrollton Ave., 504-598-5536 (Walk 17)

Vintage 329 vintage329.com, 329 Royal St., 504-525-2262

Yvonne LaFleur yvonnelafleur.com, 8131 Hampson St., 504-866-9666 (Walk 16)

MISCELLaNEOUS

Lavin-Bernick Center tulane.edu/studentaffairs/lbc, McAlister Place, 504-865-5705 (Walk 15)

Maple Street visitmaplestreet.com (Walk 16)

Ronald McDonald House rmhc-nola.org, 4403 Canal St., 504-486-6668 (Walk 17)

Royal Sonesta Hotel New Orleans sonesta.com/royalneworleans, 300 Bourbon St., 504-586-0300 (Walk 4)

Index

aBOUT THe auTHor

BARRI BRONSTON is a lifelong New Orleanian who takes every opportunity to explore the city's neighborhoods, museums, parks, restaurants, and watering holes. She graduated with a bachelor's degree in journalism from the University of Missouri and spent most of her career as a staff writer at *The Times-Picayune,* where she covered parenting, education, and other topics. She is currently assistant director of public relations at Tulane University.

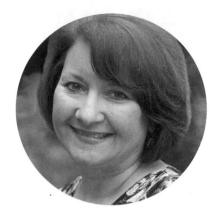

Photo: Sally Asher / Tulane University